# OUR FRAGILE BRAINS

## A CHRISTIAN PERSPECTIVE ON BRAIN RESEARCH

### D. GARETH JONES

INTER-VARSITY PRESS

*InterVarsity Press is the book-publishing division of Inter-Varsity Christian Fellowship.*

*CANADA: InterVarsity Press, 1875 Leslie St., Unit 10, Don Mills, Ontario M3B 2M5, Canada*

*GREAT BRITAIN: Inter-Varsity Press, 38 De Montfort Street, Leicester LE1 7GP, England*

*UNITED STATES: InterVarsity Press, Box F, Downers Grove, Illinois 60515*

*Various persons and publishers have granted permission to reprint figures. Acknowledgment is made on the figures themselves.*

*ISBN 0-87784-792-4*

*Printed in the United States of America*

---

**Library of Congress Cataloging in Publication Data**

*Jones, David Gareth.*
    *Our fragile brains.*

    *Bibliography: p.*
    *Includes index.*
    *1. Brain. 2. Human behavior. 3. Man (Christian theology) I. Title.*
*QP376.J58      153      80-20165*
*ISBN 0-87784-792-4*

---

| 18 | 17 | 16 | 15 | 14 | 13 | 12 | 11 | 10 | 9 | 8 | 7 | 6 | 5 | 4 | 3 | 2 | 1 |
|----|----|----|----|----|----|----|----|----|---|---|---|---|---|---|---|---|---|
| 96 | 95 | 94 | 93 | 92 | 91 | 90 | 89 | 88 | 87 | 86 | 85 | 84 | 83 | 82 | 81 | | |

# List of Figures

# Acknowledgments

*My indebtedness to various writers is evident in the pages that follow. The perspective within which their views are portrayed is my own, and I trust they have not been distorted in any way by my handling of them. Thanks are also due to Ms. Wendy Bartlett for her meticulous typing of the manuscript and to Mrs. Barbara Telfer for the preparation of the diagrams. I am especially grateful to the members of my family, who have to live with an inveterate writer: to Beryl, Kathryn, Martyn and Carolyn I say thank you.*

# 1

## Two Handfuls of Pinkish-grey Matter

THE HUMAN BRAIN is one of the most fascinating objects we are likely to study. We are fascinated with studies of the brain because we become the object of the study as well as its initiators. No book about the brain can ignore the relationship between what we are as people and the brains we possess. But once this relationship is conceded, we are confronted by an array of critical issues encompassing the nature of the relationship—the consequences for individuals of damage to their brains, the implications for human freedom and dignity of brain and behavior control, and the responsibility for providing an adequate environment in which people and their brains may develop adequately. Beyond these considerations are the more directly philosophical ones, revolving around the mind-brain paradigm, which have repercussions for our perception of reality.

A common thread throughout this diversity of issues is our view of the human person. Consequently, we shall return to that theme repeatedly. Our aim will be to view the human brain within the perspective of the human person, and the human person within the perspective of God's purposes. The emphasis will be on *wholeness,* placing aspects of brain structure and function within the context of the brain as a whole and integrating them within the framework of an individual's aspirations and fears, desires and needs.

Contemporary understanding of the brain poses a multi-pronged challenge to Christian thinking. Time and time again it forces Christians to consider just what it is they believe about human nature, about human dignity and freedom, about the extent of social control they are prepared to accept, about the status of individuals, about the validity of certain meditative and drug-induced states of altered consciousness, and about the nature of the mind and soul. Such issues are both fundamental and practical, with doctrinal and experiential repercussions. Our reaction to them, whether or not we are Christians, will have implications for our response to the challenges of present-day society. To regard these issues as a threat, from which we recoil with repulsion, will insure that we shall neither understand them nor are in a position to control them. They will control us. My plea is that we regard them not as a threat but rather as a challenge. When approached as a challenge, as I have approached them in this book, the issues force Christians to work out in a more meaningful way than before the doctrines of human nature and the human person, of freedom, dignity, responsibility, compassion and hope.

Although I write as a neuroscientist, it is my hope that this book will be seen as an exercise in applied theology as much as in neurobiology. In fact, there should be no distinction, since a holistic view of the brain demands both approaches and is incomplete without both.

## History of Ideas on the Brain

For us today it is self-evident that all thinking takes place in the brain. It is the seat of our thought processes; it is the organ responsible for consciousness, self-examination and inquiry. Nevertheless, these points were for many years the subject of ardent debate. In classical antiquity and beyond, controversy raged over the correct location of the soul, whether it was in the brain or in its principal contender for that honor, the heart. Implicit in this debate was an idea foreign to most of us, that the soul was the object of importance—and its location in the brain or heart was an interesting subsidiary matter. The soul was the life force necessary for ordinary, day-to-day existence. Both brain and heart were of lesser significance than the ephemeral soul.

The idea that the brain was the repository of the soul was first put forward in about the sixth century B.C. A little later Hippocrates committed himself in no uncertain terms to the supremacy of the brain as the source of our intellectual powers. He wrote:

Men ought to know that from the brain and the brain only arise our pleasures, joys, laughter and jests as well as our sorrows, pains, griefs and tears. . . . It is the same thing which makes us mad or delirious, inspires us with dread and fear, whether by night or by days, brings sleeplessness, inopportune mistakes, aimless anxieties, absentmindedness and acts that are contrary to habit. . . .

Despite such stirring words, Hippocrates failed to examine the brain. It was left to others such as Herophilus in the fourth century B.C. and above all to Galen about five hundred years later to gather information about the brain by examining the real thing. Their work substantiated not only that the "soul" was located somewhere in the brain but that there are motor and sensory nerves that are connected to different parts of the brain. This primitive concept proved to be a forerunner of the modern idea that specific regions of the brain are associated with specific functions.

Another major concept formulated in classical antiquity concerned the "marvelous net" or *rete mirabile* (Fig. 1.1), a small network of blood vessels. First described by Herophilus, it was incorporated by Galen (A.D. 130-200) into his

*Figure 1.1   Depiction of the human* rete mirabile *from an illustration by Walter Hermann Ryff published in 1541. Reprinted, by permission, from Edwin Clarke and Kenneth Dewhurst,* An Illustrated History of Brain Function *(1972).*

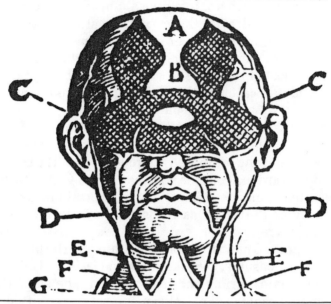

general theory of human bodily function. Galen was so influential that the *rete* was accepted as a feature of the human brain until the sixteenth century. Most observers throughout those centuries assumed that Galen had dissected human brains, whereas in reality he had studied the brains of the ox and pig, animals that have a well-developed *rete*. Human beings do not possess one. Yet on the basis of Galen's authority, most scientists throughout the Middle Ages accepted his description rather than their own observations of human brains.

Why so much emphasis on the *rete mirabile?* According to Galen, "vital spirits" were produced in the heart and distributed to all parts of the body. On reaching the cranial cavity, the blood entered that rich network of fine blood vessels at the base of the brain where the vital spirits were converted into "animal spirits." Galen, who regarded the animal spirits or "psychic pneuma" as the life force and source of all intellect, thought they were stored in the large cavities within the brain, the ventricles. From there they entered the nerves, which were regarded as hollow tubes mediating both movement and sensation. In addition, Galen, in his inconsistent way, also held that the ventricles were the site of production of animal spirits.

Thus, three fundamental concepts were formulated during classical antiquity: the location of the soul in the brain, the existence of nerves associated with the brain, and the role of the *rete mirabile* in the generation of animal spirits. A further influential idea was added during the medieval period: the *cell doctrine of brain function*. In essence, it said that mental processes occur in cells of the brain. Of course the word *cell* was being used in a totally different way from today's usage. Then, it simply denoted the ventricles of the brain. The idea that intellectual functions took place in a cavity, which seems odd to us, held sway for many years. The different ventricles were even given different functions to perform, including imagination, reasoning and memory (Fig. 1.2).

One must remember that during this time not much actual study of the brain was being carried out. Of course there were exceptions, such as Galen. His good influence, however, was largely negated over the ensuing years as his ideas took on the aura of holy writ, supplanting in the minds of medieval scientists any need to carry out further investigations. Hence errors and outmoded views were promulgated through the centuries, until a new experimental era burst into existence in the fifteenth and sixteenth centuries. We should note, however, another reason why Galen's system of thought held sway for so long: his spirit doctrine fitted in with contemporary Christian thinking on the soul. It appeared that the brain was the repository not only of thought but also of spiritual forces.

During the Renaissance, the cell doctrine began to lose ground, partly because of renewed emphasis on the struc-

Figure 1.2   Drawing of a "Disease Man" from about 1500, showing the division of the head into four compartments: common sense, imagination, rational thought, memory. Above the head is written: "The head is divided into four little cells." Reprinted, by permission, from Edwin Clarke and Kenneth Dewhurst, An Illustrated History of Brain Function (1972).

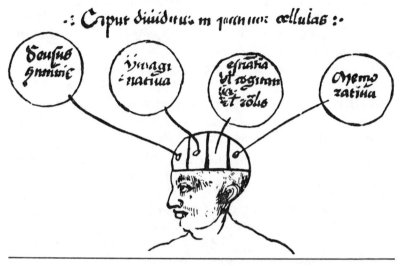

ture of the ventricles and the ventricular system. As the actual structure of the ventricles assumed a place of importance, theoretical ideas surrounding the cell doctrine receded somewhat. Observation and dissection were gradually coming into prominence, pushing the authority of Galen into the background. The many reasons for that shift in approach include an increasing emphasis on human beings rather than on God (or, in more general terms, on a dominant spiritual realm). Thus, with the emergence of Renaissance humanism, the paradigm within which scientists were working was undergoing a major change. During that time, demonstration that the ventricles contained cerebrospinal fluid discounted the likelihood that they were the seat of mental activity.

Of course the older ideas about brain function were not discarded overnight. Nevertheless, a renewed emphasis on observation was firmly established with the work of people such as Leonardo da Vinci (1452-1519) and Andreas Vesalius (1514-1564). Although their approach combined medieval physiology and Renaissance anatomy, their relatively accurate anatomy heralded the start of a new era. Their emphasis on the form and function of the ventricles as structures worthy of serious investigation had much in common with more modern scientific attitudes. In short, they were coming to depend far more on what they could observe and describe, and far less on what they thought structures *should* represent. Observation was gradually overtaking

*Figure 1.3   Drawing by Leonardo da Vinci in about 1493, comparing the layers of the scalp with an onion. The ventricles of the brain, drawn horizontally behind the eye, correspond to the description given by the old anatomists. From the Royal Library, Windsor Castle. Copyright reserved.*

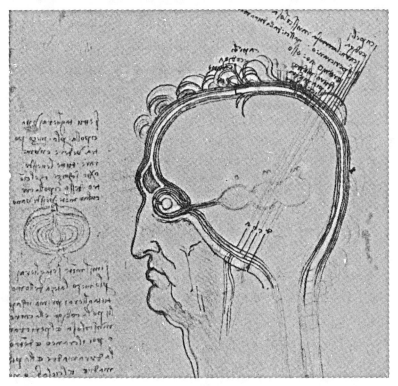

the tradition embedded in Galen.

Perhaps the supreme example of that transformation was Leonardo, the true Renaissance man who could do almost everything. He refused to believe that things could not be done simply because they had not been done before. What is particularly interesting about his anatomical studies is that some of the early ones, carried out between 1487 and 1493, were strongly influenced by traditional views. An example is his depiction of the ventricles of the brain as interconnecting spheres (Fig. 1.3).

After some fifteen years Leonardo returned to his anatomical investigations, laying great stress on actual dissec-

*Figure 1.4   Drawings by Leonardo da Vinci in about 1508. The brain had been injected with melted wax to highlight the anatomy of the cerebral ventricles. The notes in Leonardo's handwriting consist of detailed instructions on the technique of injection. Compare with Figure 1:11 for a modern view of the ventricles. From the Royal Library, Windsor Castle. Copyright reserved.*

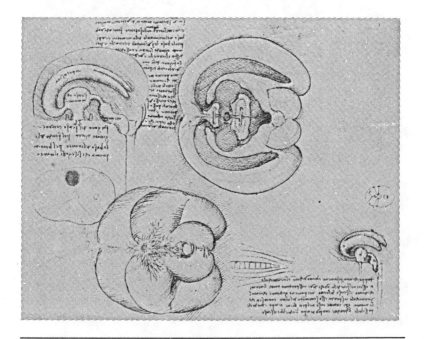

tions (both human and ox). Dissecting at least thirty bodies, he devised ingenious solutions for particular anatomical problems. He was intrigued by the ventricles of the brain and managed to demonstrate them by the injection of melted wax. The resulting wax cast of the ventricles, although slightly distorted, had a far more realistic shape (Fig. 1.4) than his earlier depiction.

In spite of such dramatic advances, people were still a long way from a modern understanding of the brain. The substance of the brain, which is what the brain is all about to most people, was largely unknown. Vesalius and another anatomist by the name of Berengario da Carpi (c. 1460-1530), however, at last put an end to the fable of the *rete mirabile* in human physiology—a small point perhaps, but a triumph for observation over tradition.

With the coming of the seventeenth century, the focus shifted from the ventricles to the cerebral hemispheres— from the cavities of the brain to the brain substance itself. What is astounding is that before the seventeenth century, the cerebral hemispheres were considered of little importance. The cerebral convolutions on the surface of the brain had been virtually ignored or depicted in an amazingly slipshod manner. They were compared to coils of intestine and were sometimes drawn just like that, even though they looked very different. The early anatomists "saw" what they thought they should see and drew what they thought they should be drawing. The fact that a large gap can exist between the external world and what people perceive applies today as much as it did then.

Outstanding figures in the seventeenth century included Franciscus de le Boë ("Sylvius," 1614-1672) and Thomas Willis (1621-1675). Sylvius suggested that the animal spirits were secreted from the cerebral and cerebellar cortices, that is, from the outer layers of the cerebral and cerebellar hemispheres. Although his view was still limited by anthropomorphic allusions, he firmly localized the higher thought processes in the brain substance. Willis was a more modern figure. Recognizing the functional importance of the cortex, he considered that other parts of the brain substance were also significant. For instance, he speculated that imagination resided in the corpus callosum, reasoning in the corpus striatum and memory in the cerebral cortex. Inadequate as these ideas appear today, Willis had broken away from the far more stultifying ideas that had previously held sway. The world of the spirits was on its way out; its replacement would be impersonal and, some might say, materialistic. But replacement had to come if the mysteries of the brain and of human thought were to be exposed to public scrutiny.

We thus arrive at a dilemma. Clearly, it is imperative to regard the brain as open to all sorts of investigations. Yet the brain is regarded as worthy of such investigations only because it is basic to what we are as persons, to our thinking, our uniqueness and our personalities. Its importance as an object of study therefore derives from our presuppositions about its significance. To treat the brain as a serious object of scientific study necessitated eliminating the world of vital spirits. Does it also lead to an elimination of the "soul," or the "mind," or any other immaterial aspect of the human person?

We shall return to that question in the final chapter. One person who needs to be mentioned at this juncture, however, is René Descartes (1596-1650). He made a radical distinction between mind and body, emphasizing the machinelike nature of the body (and hence, brain), while at the same time clinging tenaciously to an immaterial "mind." His dualism enabled him to treat the brain in as mechanistic a fashion as he wished, without compromising his views on the soul and mind. Nevertheless, Descartes's need of some point of contact between the two realms found expression in his designation of the pineal gland at the base of the brain as the location of the soul (see chapter 8).

Accurate observations and drawings obviously depend on relatively unbiased observers, those who are not tempted to prejudge too much what they will see. Given such disciplined

observers, the next step in understanding depends on research—asking the right questions and planning the right
experiments. The experimental phase in brain research
commenced in earnest at the end of the eighteenth and beginning of the nineteenth centuries, when the "science" of
*phrenology* made its debut. Devised by Franz Gall (1758-
1828) and Johann Spurzheim (1776-1832), phrenology was
based on the belief that mental and moral faculties were
located in specific areas of the brain's surface. It followed
that a surfeit or deficiency of any faculty could be detected
by examining the cranium. To convert such ideas into practical terms was relatively simple: the head was divided into
precisely defined compartments, each with its own specific
function. For example, a high forehead was a sign of intellectual ability, whereas an elongated occipital (back) region

*Figure 1.5   An example of the localization of "organs" or qualities on the surface
of the skull by phrenologists. The drawing shown here is by Franz Gall, within the
period 1810-1819, the numbers representing qualities such as friendship, cleverness,
pride and memory of words. Reprinted, by permission, from Edwin Clarke and
Kenneth Dewhurst,* An Illustrated History of Brain Function *(1972).*

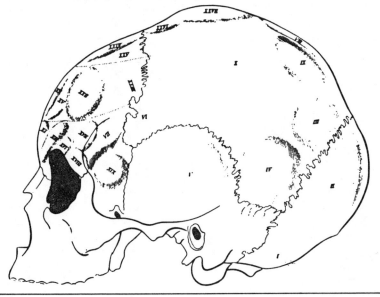

*Figure 1.6    A phrenological bust advertised in 1916 as a "new" phrenological bust with more than a hundred divisions. Reprinted, by permission, from Edwin Clarke and Kenneth Dewhurst,* An Illustrated History of Brain Function *(1972).*

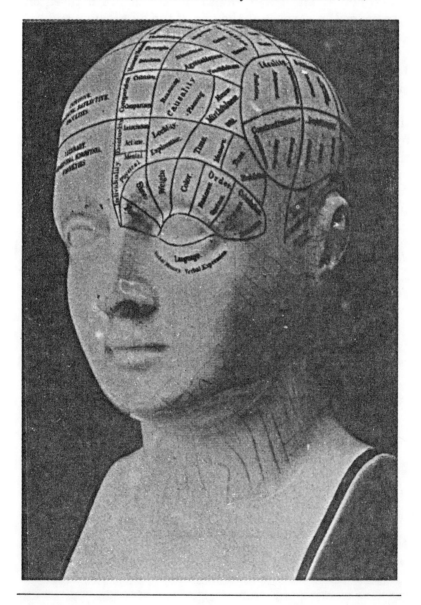

indicated loyalty and devotion. Other faculties with their own brain regions included prudence, modesty, sexual instincts, aggressiveness and so on.

Phrenology became popular and, as invariably happens, Gall's disciples were less restrained than the master himself. So, to Gall's twenty-seven mental faculties, each with its own site in the brain (Fig. 1.5), his followers added further sites and increasingly complex arrangements until the enthusiasm of some brought the whole movement into disrepute (Fig. 1.6).

Phrenology is intriguing because, although it was basically unscientific, it had useful elements in it. In fact it was close enough to being correct to render it of value to science; Gall himself had carried out some respectable anatomical investigations into the structure of the cerebral hemispheres. Phrenology was also of value in turning people away from too rigid an adherence to the concept of the Cartesian soul (with its implicit dualism) toward a view of the brain in which material and mechanical functions are paramount.

Unfortunately, phrenology was essentially incorrect in the nature of the localization it postulated in the brain, and hence was misleading. It had to be discredited before further advance could take place. That was accomplished by Pierre Flourens in the 1820s. As a result of studies of stimulation of the brain as well as removal of small portions of it, Flourens suggested that intellectual and perceptual functions were represented diffusely throughout the cerebral hemispheres rather than confined to the surface. Although his observations were erroneous, he succeeded in toppling phrenology. In 1870 Gustav Fritsch and Edward Hitzig succeeded in actually localizing various functions, including motor ones, in specific areas of the brain, thereby ushering in the modern era of cortical localization. A few years before, in 1861, a French surgeon, Pierre-Paul Broca, had a patient with a speech deficiency. After the patient's death, Broca noted a lesion in the left hemisphere of the brain and proposed that the affected region might be a center for speech—another early example of cortical localization (see chapter 2).

Our historical review can end here as we are now close enough to a modern view of the brain. The brain has been established as the fundamental regulator of our personalities and mental attributes. Moreover, from a scientific viewpoint, the most profitable way of approaching it is to regard it as an entity capable of description and understanding in mechanical terms. That understanding necessitates an experimental approach, making judicious use of animal models where required to extend our knowledge of the human brain.

To appreciate some of the issues surrounding the brain requires a basic understanding of its organization and functioning. In order to provide that essential groundwork the next section will summarize the way the brain presents itself to us as an integral part of our anatomical selves.

## The Brain as a System

The brain is just one part of the nervous system, albeit a very important part and the one of principal concern in this book. Together with the spinal cord the brain forms the *central nervous system* (CNS), situated centrally within our bodies. By contrast, the *peripheral nervous system* (PNS) has a peripheral location and consists of a large number of nerves (Fig. 1.7), including those running in our arms and legs. Such nerves connect the outlying parts of the body with the spinal cord. What is called the *autonomic nervous system* (ANS) is more difficult to understand because it has nerves originating from within both the central and peripheral nervous systems. It can be referred to as the involuntary nervous system, since its chief function is to regulate bodily organs without any active (or voluntary) help. Among the most important organs thus regulated are the heart and lungs. Our involuntary system helps us adjust both to the environment inside our bodies and to the external environment.

Nerves of the peripheral nervous system send messages to and from the spinal cord. *Afferent* nerves run toward the cord and *efferent* ones away from it. Afferent nerves, therefore, keep the brain and spinal cord in touch with the remainder of the body and with the world outside the body. Efferent nerves convey messages to the body's muscles, making it possible for the brain, and hence the person, to respond to the world outside the body (Fig. 1.7). Thus the afferent

*Figure 1.7   Diagram to show the relation of the brain and spinal cord, constituting the central nervous system, to some of the nerves making up the peripheral nervous system.*

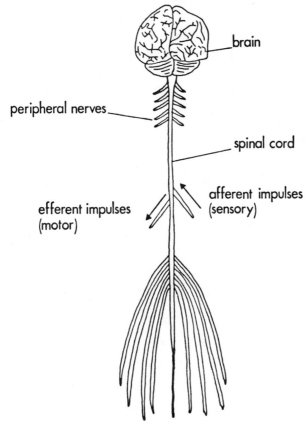

nerves are *sensory,* conveying information about sensations of the body into the spinal cord. The efferent or *motor* nerves trigger the movements of muscles, bringing into action arms, hands and legs.

When an object such as the pen I am using comes into contact with the skin, messages travel along afferent (sensory) nerves to the spinal cord. The nerves end in the so-called *grey matter* of the spinal cord, a butterfly-shaped area consisting of large nerve cells (Fig. 1.8). The messages are then passed to other nerve cells which send long fibers upward in the outer *white matter* of the cord. In that way the messages reach not only many parts of the spinal cord but also the brain.

The long nerve fibers traveling upward in the cord are bunched together as the *ascending tracts,* which carry to the brain all the information from the whole body, with the exception of information from the head (eyes, ears and so on). The brain decides on a course of action and sends the appropriate message back along the spinal cord via the *descending tracts,* also found in the cord's white matter (Fig. 1.8). They

*Figure 1.8    Section through the lumbar region of the spinal cord. The descending tract comes from the motor cortex of the brain; the ascending tract terminates in the thalamus and sensory cortex within the brain.*

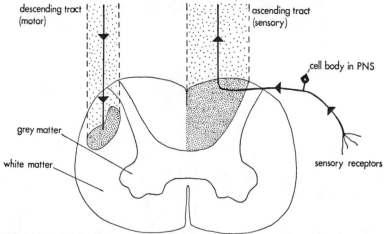

convey the brain's response to the required level of the cord. From that point the message is carried via an efferent (motor) nerve which, in turn, activates appropriate muscles to move in the manner dictated by the brain.

The brain, thus kept in touch with events in its environment, is able to respond on the basis of information stores it has built up over the individual's lifetime. The brain is able to remember and also to learn, because whenever its response is inappropriate for a given situation the response is modified on a subsequent occasion.

*Figure 1.9  View of the human brain from the left side, showing its subdivision into forebrain, midbrain and hindbrain. The smaller convolutions on the surface of the brain are not depicted.*

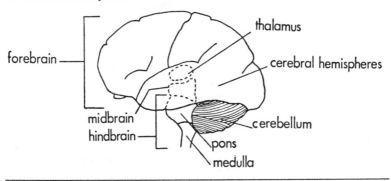

Figure 1.9 shows the human brain subdivided into three principal regions: forebrain, midbrain and hindbrain. The forebrain consists of the cerebral hemispheres and the more deeply situated thalamus. The hindbrain consists of the pons, medulla and cerebellum. In another commonly used descriptive scheme, the brain's major components are the cerebrum, brain stem and cerebellum; the cerebrum consists essentially of the cerebral hemispheres and the brain stem accounts for everything else except the cerebellum.

The *forebrain*, the region we shall focus on primarily, consists largely of the *cerebral hemispheres*—one on either side, joined together across the midline by a bundle of fibers

*Figure 1.10    Vertical section of the human brain in the midline, displaying medial views of many brain regions.*

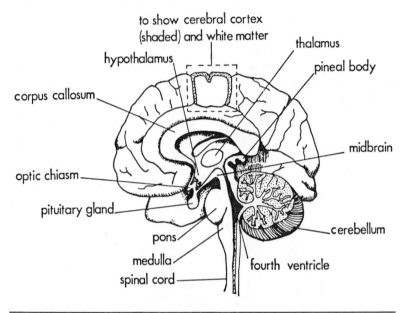

known as the *corpus callosum* (Fig. 1.10). Each hemisphere consists of a core of white matter and a thin enveloping rind of grey matter, 3-4 mm thick, an arrangement opposite to that found in the spinal cord. The peripheral grey matter in the brain is known as the *cerebral cortex.*

The surface of the hemispheres is far from smooth. Its many fissures are called the *sulci,* the folds between them the *gyri.* The great irregularity in the adult increases considerably the surface area of the hemispheres and therefore the area of the cerebral cortex. At birth the irregularity is already present, although the sulci are relatively shallow.

The cerebral cortex contains many millions of nerve cell bodies, densely packed together. The underlying white matter is largely constructed from nerve fibers. The cortex is concerned with conscious behavior and with such "higher" activities as learning, memory and the coding of the individual's experiences. Yet the hemispheres are *not* absolutely essential to life; at least a few months of existence with basic respiratory and excretory functions are possible without them. Anything resembling normal human life is, however, impossible without them.

Deeply embedded within each cerebral hemisphere is the oval-shaped *thalamus* (Fig. 1.10), the chief function of which is to relay sensory information from the spinal cord's ascending tracts to the cerebral cortex. In other words, the thalamus is the final relay station where ascending, sensory influences are processed before being transmitted to the sensory region of the cerebral cortex.

The *midbrain,* by far the smallest subdivision of the brain, is made up essentially of bundles of nerve fibers on their way up to the forebrain or down to the hindbrain. These fibers run through the *cerebral peduncles* connecting the midbrain to the cerebral hemispheres. In the remainder of the midbrain are areas associated with some aspects of hearing and sight.

The *hindbrain,* the most posterior part of the brain, is continuous with the upper end of the spinal cord (Fig. 1.9 and 1.10). It consists of the *medulla oblongata,* the *pons* and on either side of these the *cerebellum.* In this region of the brain many bundles of nerve fibers cross over the midline from right to left and vice versa. Consequently many individual fibers *decussate* (cross) in some part of the hindbrain: the pons carries fibers from one side of the cerebellum to the other, and in the *pyramids* of the medulla some tracts running between the forebrain and spinal cord cross over. That decussation of fibers is responsible for the fact that the right side of the brain, for example, controls the left side of the body. Although we are not aware of that odd arrangement during the normal course of events, it becomes obvious when something goes wrong with one side of the brain, such as a tumor growing or a blood clot cutting off the supply of blood. Symptoms affecting the left side of the body are indicative of a malfunction in the right side of the brain (probably the right cerebral hemisphere). The hindbrain as a whole is responsible for keeping the body alive as long as food and drink are provided. The cerebellum adjusts muscular tone so that upright, steady walking is possible.

Historically, much interest centered on the ventricles, which will not feature much in the remainder of our account. Together they form the ventricular system, the function of which is to produce cerebrospinal fluid and circulate it within and around the brain and spinal cord. The CNS is thus bathed in a fluid environment, and hence to some extent is protected from external injury. The form of the ventricular system is shown in Figure 1.11: the lateral ventricles lying within the cerebral hemispheres, the third ventricle close to the thalamus, and the fourth ventricle within the pons and medulla. The ventricles are interconnected by small channels, with the whole system connecting with what is called the *sub arachnoid space* around the brain and spinal cord.

*Figure 1.11   Diagram of the ventricular system, showing the location of its constituent parts within the brain. The aqueduct is a channel connecting the third and fourth ventricles.*

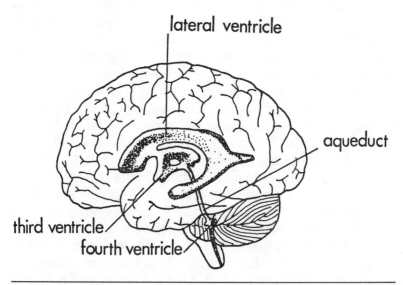

Blockage within that system leads to one form or another of *hydrocephalus,* a swelling of the ventricular system and compression of parts of the brain tissue.

## The Cerebral Hemispheres

With the general arrangement of the brain in mind, we now return to the forebrain and in particular to the cerebral hemispheres. From the side, each can be seen to consist of a number of well-defined regions, termed lobes. Recognizable on the surface are the *frontal* lobe at the front, the *occipital* at the back, and the *parietal* and *temporal* at the side with the parietal above the temporal (Fig. 1.12). Several important *fissures* (or sulci), especially the central and lateral sulci, are landmarks helpful in distinguishing one lobe from another.

Within, or related to, the structural subdivisions are areas

*Figure 1.12   Left cerebral hemisphere of the human brain showing the major lobes into which it is subdivided.*

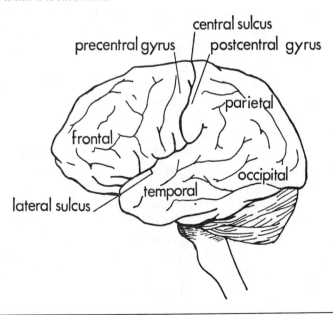

associated with particular functions; that is, the hemispheres can be subdivided into *functionally distinct regions.* Knowledge about the functional organization of the cerebral hemispheres has come from observing the effects of brain injury or disease on behavior and, more recently, from electrical stimulation of different regions of the cerebral cortex during surgery. In that way neurologists have been able to construct fairly precise maps of the hemispheres. In the 1930s, Wilder Penfield (1891-1976), a Canadian neurosurgeon, pioneered studies on the temporal lobes of human patients during operations for epileptic and other brain disorders. Because brain operations can be carried out under local anesthesia, patients are able to recount their feelings following stimulation of different brain regions.

The best-established data relate to localization of *sensory* and *motor* functions. The main motor area is the *precentral gyrus,* situated just in front of the central sulcus. The main sensory area is the *postcentral gyrus,* found just behind the central sulcus (Fig. 1.12).

When the brain of a human patient is stimulated with a small electrode during a brain operation, the patient experiences certain consequences. For example, stimulation of the precentral gyrus results in the movement of certain groups of muscles, hence its designation the motor cortex. The groups of muscles affected depend on the part of the precentral gyrus stimulated. Similarly, an injury to a part of the precentral gyrus leads to the paralysis of muscles. Thus an injury to the upper part of the gyrus leads to paralysis of the leg on the opposite side of the body; damage to the lower part of the gyrus leads to paralysis of the head and tongue. In other words, the body is represented upside down in this gyrus. Further, the parts of the body are *unequally* represented, in that the largest areas are devoted not to the largest parts of the body but to regions responsible for intricate and important movements such as those of the hands, vocal apparatus and tongue (Fig. 1.13).

To the postcentral gyrus, the principal sensory area,

*Figure 1.13  Localization of functionally distinct areas in the left cerebral hemisphere. Within the motor area, the letters represent muscle groups from different parts of the body: A, toes-knee; B, hip-wrist; C, hand; D, fingers; E, forehead-eye; F, face-lips; G, lower jaw; H, tongue-larynx-pharynx. Regions F-H are concerned with voice production.*

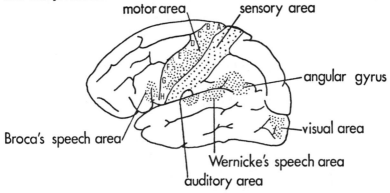

are conveyed sensations from the skin, stomach, heart, and so on; in other words, afferent impulses arising from touch, pain and heat are transformed into conscious sensations in this part of the cerebral hemispheres. Again the body is represented upside down, with greater emphasis placed on bodily regions where sensation is important, such as the lips and mouth.

*Visual* input to the cerebral cortex from the eyes goes principally to the occipital lobe where it is transformed into visual sensations (Fig. 1.13). The pathway to the visual cortex from the retinae of the eyes is a complicated one, with crossing-over of about 50 per cent of the fibers. The *auditory* area concerned with hearing lies in the temporal gyrus just within the lips of the lateral sulcus. The *olfactory* area lies on the medial aspect of each hemisphere in an area known as the *uncus*. Other areas correspond to taste, touch and pressure, and to vestibular sensations from the inner ear concerned with the positioning of the body in space.

The two major speech areas, Broca's and Wernicke's areas (Fig. 1.13), are named after the men who first suggested their significance; in both cases damage to the areas brought them to the attention of neurologists. Damage to Broca's area results in a .disturbance of language, an *aphasia,* because the muscles responsible for speech production are affected. Speech is slow and labored, although the patient can understand the speech of others. Wernicke's aphasia is quite different; superficially the speech may sound quite normal, but it lacks content and may incorporate incorrect words. The differences coincide with the location of the areas: Broca's alongside the motor region, Wernicke's between the auditory and visual areas.

For any sort of language to be produced, the two areas must be connected to each other, as well as to the auditory and visual areas. The angular gyrus shown in Figure 1.13 connects Wernicke's area to the visual cortex and therefore plays an essential role in converting a visual stimulus into an auditory one. Language and its representation will be dealt with more fully in chapter 2.

The speech areas are found in the left cerebral hemisphere (Fig. 1.13) in 96-98 per cent of the population. Consequently, the left hemisphere is conventionally referred to as the dominant (major) hemisphere, the right as the nondominant (minor) one.

In spite of continuing neurological research, large regions of the cortex are still unaccounted for. Since the major part of the cortex does not appear to have any function, people used to refer to the unassigned areas as the silent areas. Undoubtedly, that is an oversimplification. After all, our description so far has hardly touched on the myriad components of thought or of subtle behavioral changes.

Considerable attention has been paid of late to differences between the left and right hemispheres. Even in many left-handed people, the right hemisphere is the minor one. In general, the dominant hemisphere is specialized in respect to fine imaginative details, while the minor hemisphere is more concerned with organizing visuo-spatial perception, that is, with the ability to locate our bodies accurately in space. A detailed account of those differences will be given in chapter 2, along with a discussion of how the two hemispheres function as an integral unit.

Our description of the two hemispheres fails to account for a number of essential features of human existence which, one suspects, must reside in the organization of the brain. Among them are attributes such as motivation, the determination to get things done, the maintenance of a high level of interest in life around us. The operation known as *frontal leucotomy* (chapter 4), which in its classical form was in vogue in the 1940s and '50s, consisted of cutting the nerve fibers connecting the frontal lobes to the remainder of the brain. Although severe depression and excruciating pain were frequently alleviated, many patients ended up as vegetables. Their condition did not result from any loss of muscular or sensory functions; the patients simply lost all interest in themselves and their surroundings. Their last condition often was worse than the first—not because deep depression is good, but because lack of motivation is even worse. Therein lies one of the conundrums of human existence. The frontal lobes constitute the apparatus essential for regulating the state of activity of the brain. They have the function of forming stable plans and intentions capable of controlling a person's conscious behavior. In short, they are intimately concerned with the general regulation of behavior, orienting it to the future as well as to the present.

We end our account of the cerebral hemispheres with a note on the temporal lobes (Fig. 1.12). We have already seen that some of the left temporal lobe is devoted to the production of speech. Penfield's stimulation studies in the 1930s suggested that the remainder of that lobe and the contralateral one are devoted to interpretation of present experience in the light of past experience. For that reason those lobes constitute the *interpretive cortex.*

During surgical treatment of patients suffering from epileptic seizures originating in the temporal lobe, Penfield noted that electrical stimulation of the interpretive cortex occasionally produced flashbacks in which the patient re-lived an experience of an earlier period in life. In one such example, a mother, on cortical stimulation, was aware of being in her kitchen listening to the voice of her little boy who was playing outside in the yard. She was aware of neighborhood noises, such as passing cars, that might mean danger to him. It is quite likely that what was being stim-ulated in such instances was the *hippocampus,* a long twisted structure lying deep within the temporal cortex (Fig. 4.4).

Up to this point everything described has been visible with the naked eye. Observations at such a level have severe limitations: they provide no information about the tissues and cells making up the brain. For further under-standing of brain function a microscope is necessary. A light microscope magnifies up to 2,000 times, but for some purposes an electron microscope, which enables us to view images up to at least 200 thousand times greater than their actual dimensions, is even more useful.

### The World of the Nerve Cells

Most nerve cells of the brain are found in the cerebral hemi-spheres and, in particular, in its outer layer of grey matter, the cerebral cortex. The human cerebral cortex contains something like $10^{10}$ to $10^{14}$ nerve cells. With that astro-nomical number of basic units, the cerebral cortex is some-times referred to as the "great analyzer." If there are a minimum of $10^{10}$ nerve cells in the cerebral cortex, that number, 10 billion, is about 2.5 times the human population of the earth. Imagine three planets with the same population as the earth, with telegraph and radio links between every group of people on those planets. With that in mind, one begins to envision the type of situation present in the brain of each individual.

That is only a start, however. Each nerve cell makes contact with some 5,000 or so other nerve cells; that is, each nerve cell has up to 5,000 junctions with neighboring nerve

*Figure 1.14  Illustration of the large number of synaptic connections between one nerve cell and processes of other nerve cells.*

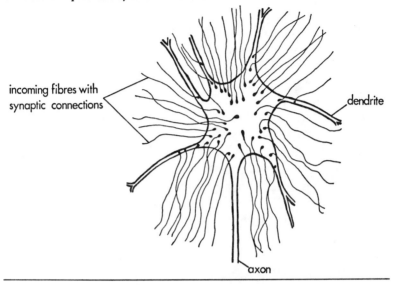

incoming fibres with synaptic connections

dendrite

axon

cells, some as many as 50,000 junctions (Fig. 1.14). At those *synaptic junctions* or *synapses,* information is passed between the nerve cells. What is significant about that process is that the information may be modified during its transfer. The number of sites at which information may be altered in some way is, therefore, astronomical, since the number of synaptic junctions within just a gram of brain tissue is of the order of $4 \times 10^{11}$. The brain's cellular organization shows an almost unbelievable profusion of *connections* between nerve cells. Without such intricate connectivity, learning processes would be impossible.

Thus the number of connections within *one* human brain rivals the number of stars and galaxies in the universe and far exceeds the human population of our planet. It is obvious that the information potential of even one brain is formidable. But the brains of all individuals differ in their interconnections, so that the problem of understanding *individual* brains in depth—as opposed to *the* brain—

takes on unexpected dimensions.

By using a combination of stains and preparative techniques it has been possible to work out the structure of individual nerve cells and their interrelationships. Although much work remains to be done, we owe an immense debt to the pioneering studies in the late nineteenth century and the early years of this century by people such as Camillo Golgi (1843-1926) and Santiago Ramón y Cajal (1852-1934).

Each nerve cell consists of three regions: a *cell body* containing the nucleus; an *axon,* which is a long single process (extension) conducting impulses *away* from the cell body; and several short processes, the *dendrites,* which increase the surface area of the nerve cell and conduct impulses *toward* the cell body (Fig. 1.15). Axons vary in length from a fraction of a millimeter to several meters. They

*Figure 1.15 Diagrammatic representation of a complete nerve cell (left), an enlargement of one of its dendritic branches (center), and a further enlargement of the point of synaptic contact between a spine of that dendrite and a neighboring nerve cell (right).*

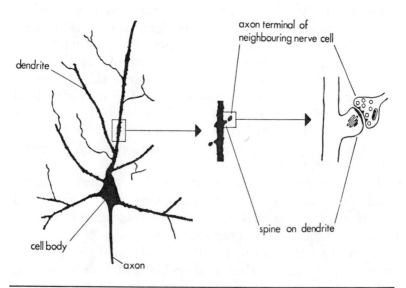

also vary in diameter, the larger ones conducting impulses more rapidly than the smaller ones. The dendrites branch extensively, like the trunk of a tree, enabling any one nerve cell to make contact with, and so receive impulses from, large numbers of other nerve cells.

A nerve functions basically like a telephone wire, conducting electrical impulses or messages rapidly over long distances. Inside and outside the nerve fiber are salt solutions, separated from one another only by the nerve-cell membrane. In the resting state the solution within the fiber has a high concentration of potassium ions and a low concentration of sodium ions; the solution surrounding the fiber has the opposite, a high concentration of sodium ions and a low concentration of potassium ions. Since the two solutions contain electrolytes they are capable of conducting an electric current. To complete the picture, the fluid outside the fiber contains calcium ions and both solutions contain chloride ions.

When an impulse passes along a nerve fiber, the resistance of the nerve membrane surrounding the fiber decreases, thereby increasing its permeability to sodium ions. Sodium ions pass into the fiber, making the inside of the membrane more positive. At much the same time there is a compensatory outflow of potassium ions.

Those events cause a "wave" of what is termed potential change to be conducted along the fiber as neighboring areas are excited, and an *action potential* is propagated. Each cycle of events affects an extremely small area of membrane, and the passage of the impulse is in one direction only. Further, another impulse cannot follow until the events connected with the previous one have been concluded. That fixes the number of impulses a nerve can carry in a given time. Once a nerve impulse has started, it is self-propagating throughout the length of that fiber.

Impulse propagation occurs along the whole length of a nerve fiber, both axon and dendrites. At the end of the fiber an impulse arrives at a junction between nerve cells, that is, at a synapse; a different method of conduction is responsible for transmitting an impulse to the adjacent nerve cell, making use of chemical transmitter substances.

Since the only message carried by nerves is an *electrochemical* one, all the body's dealings with both its internal and external environments have to be translated into that electrochemical "language" to be conveyed to and from the control centers. To begin to grasp the way the brain works, we must also explore it at that level. To gain much information about the junctional regions between nerve cells, however, a technical breakthrough was required. It came with the invention of the *electron microscope* in the late 1930s, although such instruments were not applied to biological work in a serious way until the early 1950s. For most practical purposes in biology, magnifications in the range of 20,000-100,000 times are routinely used; even that magnification introduces a completely different dimension from that of light microscopy.

Basically, a synapse consists of three parts: the *presynaptic* terminal, the *postsynaptic* terminal and, between them, a gap or *cleft* (Fig. 1.16). By the turn of the century, neurohistologists had decided that neurons were separate units rather than integral parts of a network or reticulum. The distinct gap thus expected at each synaptic junction was eventually demonstrated by electron micrographs; the presynaptic terminal belongs to one neuron, the postsynaptic to another, with a clear gap separating them. In fact the presynaptic terminal is the enlarged ending of an *axon* and the postsynaptic terminal is usually either a *dendrite* or *cell body*. Impulses travel along the axon toward the synapse, stimulating or inhibiting the postsynaptically located dendrite or cell body (Fig. 1.15).

Within the presynaptic terminal are some small, usually spherical structures termed *synaptic vesicles,* plus one or more *mitochondria* which provide energy for the transmission process. In addition, some dense projections appearing as triangular profiles represent modifications of the

*Figure 1.16   Diagram of the structure of a synapse, as seen at very high magnification in the electron microscope.*

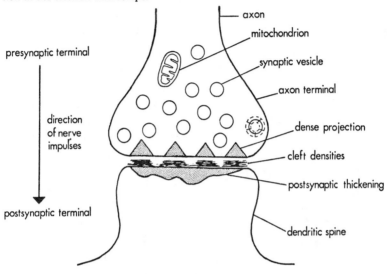

presynaptic membrane. When an impulse arrives at a synaptic terminal, it triggers off the release of a chemical substance, or transmitter (generally either acetylcholine or noradrenaline), carried by the synaptic vesicles to the presynaptic membrane. After being discharged into the cleft and diffusing across the cleft, the transmitter combines with receptor sites on the postsynaptic membrane. Thus information is transferred from one nerve cell to another.

Academic as "synaptic transmission" may sound, it is actually close to the reality of our everyday lives. That is because the synapse is the principal location where messages in the nervous system can be modified, and because evidence is accumulating that large numbers of drugs act at synapses (chapter 5). The synapse is thus not immune to the forces of society, nor is society free from the consequences of research on the synapse. Neurochemists are just beginning to uncover the vast potential of synaptic modification. That news may come as a ray of hope to those afflicted by certain mental disorders—but as a dire warning to those who look on any form of brain manipulation with horror.

## The Christian Stake in Brain Control

Even our cursory glimpse at the brain in this chapter shows how study of the brain can raise philosophical, theological, ethical and educational issues. Such study therefore has implications for Christian thinking, largely because of the question of human responsibility. Christian apologist and neuroscientist Donald MacKay argues that brain research introduces the issue of human responsibility at two levels: in our responsibility to explore the mysterious richness of the brain, and in our willingness to face up to the implications of brain research for our concept of human responsibility itself. Christians should be particularly interested in the brain; knowledge of the brain is linked in an intrinsic way to brain control. Even at an early stage in our discussion there can be no escape from a fundamental predicament: increased understanding of brain organization is intimately associated with power over the brains of other individuals. Given the former, the latter will follow. To construct the ethical superstructure necessary to such scientific research, Christians should be applying biblically based ethical principles. We must face up to the potential consequences of brain control and to ways in which it can be put to good effect in society.

Rigorous thinking is required. The issue of control is just the beginning. It ushers in questions about our view of human nature: our relationship to God, our sinfulness, our finitude and the extent to which we can be biologically and spiritually changed, the relationship of individuals to the demands of society, the nature of personal identity and its dependence on the structural integrity of the brain, and the relationship between present existence with its reliance on an adequately functioning brain and a future existence lacking any such reliance. Beyond all such considerations, however, is a far more immediate one: all studies of the brain, like all dealings with our fellow human beings, are to be motivated by compassion. In that context MacKay comments, "Each advance in our knowledge of brain processes is to be welcomed in principle as enhancing our sensitivity to one another's vulnerabilities, as increasing our respect for one another's strengths, and as extending our capacities to do one another good."

Study of the brain, therefore, brings us face-to-face with ourselves. Major advances in our understanding of the brain may have come from applying the relatively objective approach of science, but we can arrive at a view of our place in the world only by the use of our brains. It is impossible to separate our knowledge of the brain as a subject of interest from what we are as people. We use brains to study brains, and we are what we are because of the brains we possess.

The emphasis of this book is that we cannot with impunity isolate brains from persons. Study of the brain precipitates us into questions of the value we place on human life and the value of the aspirations of individuals, religious issues of deep concern to Christians. Moreover, the sort of control we endeavor to exert over people and their brains will depend in large measure on our beliefs about human nature. Our presuppositions play a vital role in our attitudes even when the presuppositions are not acknowledged.

If human beings are thought of as machines, there will be a tendency to treat them as machinery to be "tinkered with" and modified at will. This book will demonstrate that the brain, our most mechanistic and vulnerable part, easily lends itself to manipulation. Any guidelines for manipulation, however, must be imposed from outside; machines do not incorporate guidelines. This immense problem is an embarrassment for any purely mechanistic school of thought; yet a viable alternative is available.

Human beings may not be treated as machines. Indeed, the Christian says that they are anything but machines. They are persons who find themselves in a meaningful universe. Admittedly, there are many ways in which a human being can be *compared to* a machine; for some scientific purposes, that is a useful procedure. In the end, though, such an approach tells us little about *human* nature and aspirations. It leaves unanswered the question about *who* human beings are.

Humanity must be seen in the context of a universe incorporating values and based on values. In other words, we are looking for a view of human beings which sees them as having value because they are an integral part of a value-based world. Such is the Christian view of humanity, according to which we live in a world designed and upheld by God, to whom we have personal meaning. Each individual fits into a God-centered system and achieves meaning and individuality within that framework.

With such a base we can see not only that man *in toto* has meaning, but that every aspect of human makeup and life also has significance. That is why it is impossible to isolate anyone's brain or personality from his or her existence as a person. It is tantalizingly easy to confuse a person's brain or its array of psychological manifestations with the person. Whenever that happens, we have confused claims about brains with claims about people. We need to remember that people think and make decisions, not brains.

Discussions about the brain should not be isolated from discussions about the people who possess those brains or the society in which the people live or their relationships to each other and to God. Whatever contributes to our being must be seen in the context of our relationship to God as well as to our fellow creatures. All of us are created by one and the same God to live out our lives in harmony and responsible community. It is dangerous to think that society has no responsibility for the way in which one person treats the brain of another. We are profoundly responsible for each other, including each other's integrity as human persons.

Christians should be alert to the whole realm of brain control out of a serious concern for the integrity of human beings as people. That challenge will emerge in a number of different ways in the forthcoming chapters, its details worked out in relation to specific issues. What should emerge is a sense of the intimate relationship between the state of people's brains and the quality of their lives.

# 2

## Language and Consciousness

IN OUR DISCUSSION of general features of the human brain, speech centers were mentioned. They represent the structural and functional basis of language, which has traditionally been regarded as the supreme distinguishing feature of humanity. We will now consider the speech centers in detail and the extent to which language is indeed confined to human beings.

### Language and Its Production

Language is an immensely significant means of communication between individuals. Its potential far surpasses that of signals based on olfactory, tactile, visual and auditory cues, providing a means whereby a very large number of signals can be combined to produce words and combinations of words. Language is essential for the elaboration of abstract concepts, the invention of new ideas, and the attempts of human beings to understand themselves and their world. It enables an individual to learn from a variety of other individuals and not solely from parents. Hence a suprahereditary form of cultural "inheritance" is introduced into human experience.

But is language found only in humans? What about the nonhuman primates? In the seventeenth century René Descartes argued that use of language was the critical factor distinguishing *Homo sapiens* from the beasts. In 1637 Descartes wrote: "For it is a very remarkable thing that there are no men, not even the insane, so dull and stupid that they cannot put words together in a manner to convey their thoughts. On the contrary, there is no other animal however perfect and fortunately situated it may be, that can do the same." In contrast, the eighteenth-century physician, Julian La Mettrie, denied that language is a uniquely human feature, contending instead that any nonhuman linguistic deficits may be due to such causes as impoverished environment or lack of proper training.

In the latter part of the seventeenth century, John Locke contended that nonhuman animals are incapable of thinking in abstract terms. An Irish philosopher and bishop, George Berkeley, replied that if so, many of those that pass for men must be reckoned into their number. Do we yet know whether any nonhuman primates are capable of abstract thought—in any degree?

Over the past century or so, repeated attempts have been made to teach chimpanzees to perform tasks of which humans are capable. Many ethological studies investigated the extent of cooperation, foresight, future planning and even deception in chimpanzees' behavior patterns. Specific efforts at teaching chimpanzees to speak concentrated until recent years on raising young chimps in an experimenter's own household alongside a young baby. Everything needed by the growing child was duplicated for the chimpanzee, so that in effect there were two children. After three years or so the two were compared. Inevitably the end result was the same. Although the three-year-old chimp far outstripped the three-year-old child in manual dexterity, the language capabilities of the child were blossoming forth in contrast with a few stuttering "words" of the chimp. From such attempts it was widely and reasonably concluded that language is beyond chimpanzees, since they appeared incapable of anything remotely resembling competent, communicative speech. Before pursuing that issue further, however, we should look at the anatomical features of the human brain that make speech possible.

We have already mentioned that the first hints of the existence of speech centers were provided by examination of damaged brains. It was in 1861 that French physician Pierre-Paul Broca recognized that damage to a specific region of the brain resulted in a language disturbance. That (posterior-inferior) region of the frontal lobe, subsequently named *Broca's area* (Fig. 2.1), is located close to the part of the motor cortex controlling muscles of the face, jaw, tongue, palate and larynx.

In 1865 Broca noted that disorders of language occurred only when that area of the *left* hemisphere was damaged. Equivalent damage in the right hemisphere has no effect on

*Figure 2.1 Left cerebral hemisphere outlining the speech centers (Broca's and Wernicke's areas) plus other brain regions implicated in the production of language.*

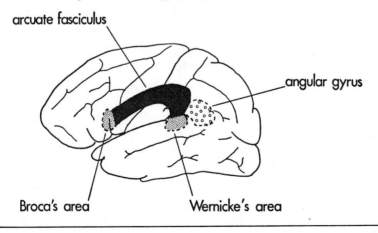

arcuate fasciculus

angular gyrus

Broca's area

Wernicke's area

linguistic abilities. Subsequent studies have confirmed Broca's early observations; 96-98 per cent of patients with permanent language disorders from brain lesions have left-hemisphere damage. Those findings led to the concept of cerebral dominance, with the left hemisphere emerging as the dominant hemisphere in a very large proportion of the population.

The aphasia resulting from damage of Broca's area is a *motor aphasia* associated with the actual *production* of language. Patients with that type of aphasia have a slow, labored speech. The style is described as telegraphic, small words and the endings of words being omitted. Asked about a trip he has taken, a patient may simply reply, "Europe . . ." Encouraged to say more, he may manage, "Go . . . Europe." This kind of faltering language and difficulty with grammatical phrases may lead an observer to the conclusion that the patient cannot understand language. That conclusion is incorrect; the block is almost entirely one of expression.

Damage to Broca's area does not invariably lead to that end-result, however. For instance, the many frontal leucotomies carried out in the 1940s and '50s must have at least injured Broca's area, yet evidently none of those patients suffered from aphasia. One surgeon removed Broca's area from both hemispheres of two patients who had not talked for more than twenty years. The amazing result was that both patients began to talk following the operation and continued to do so for many years. An intact Broca's area cannot be essential for normal speech, therefore, although a malfunctioning Broca's area may disrupt normal speech.

Thirteen years after the initial description of Broca's aphasia, a significant paper was published by a twenty-six-year-old neurologist in Breslau named Carl Wernicke. He described a lesion in the posterior-superior part of the temporal lobe (Fig. 2.1), producing an aphasia that differed from that described by Broca. In *Wernicke's aphasia* speech is rapid; it is grammatically correct, and superficially it may sound quite normal. But it has little content and frequently utilizes incorrect words or circumlocutory phrases in place of single words. Further, Wernicke's aphasia is accompanied by a *loss of understanding*.

The two centers bearing their discoverers' names by themselves are not sufficient for the production of language. They must be connected to each other by a bundle of nerve fibers, the *arcuate fasciculus* (Fig. 2.1). Yet even that connection is insufficient because both vision and hearing play an implicit role in speech. The *angular gyrus* connecting the visual cortex to Wernicke's speech center is critical in converting a visual stimulus into an appropriate auditory form. A number of sequences (depending on whether a word is heard or read) can be postulated on the basis of ideas originally put forward by Wernicke himself, as illustrated in Figure 2.2.

It is thus possible to predict the site of a brain lesion from the nature of a language disorder. A person may be able to hear a word but not speak, or hear a word but not spell it. Others with no difficulty in reading may be incapable of saying what they have read.

*Figure 2.2  Possible sequences of brain events in language. The sequences vary depending on whether a word is heard or read and on whether the response is to be spoken or written.*

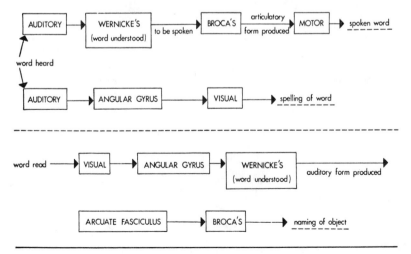

*Figure 2.3  Models showing the relationship between various language and associated disorders and the brain regions damaged in each instance.*

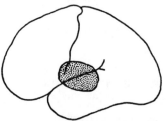

**a  communicative disability**

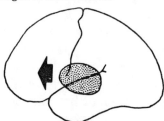

**b  expressive**

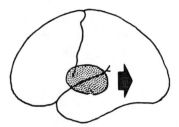

**c  confusion**

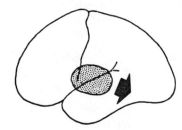

**d  reading difficulties (alexia)**

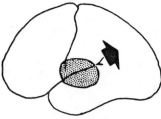

**e  semantic difficulties**

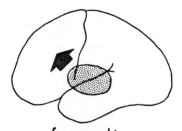

**f  agraphia**

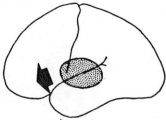

**g  dysarthria**

Viewing aphasia from an overall perspective, as Karl Pribram and other investigators, we emerge with a model like Figure 2.3. Damage to Wernicke's area results in a communicative disability in the use of language (a). When the lesion extends forward the disability becomes more expressive corresponding to a Broca type of lesion (b). When the lesion extends backward, there is confusion concerning what is to be expressed (c). A lesion running backward and downward will probably produce reading difficulties *(alexia)* because of damage to the visual region (d). The complementary lesion to (d), that is, backward and upward into the parietal cortex, will result in impairment in grasping relationships (e). An upward lesion running forward implicates the hand area of the motor cortex, so that writing difficulties *(agraphia)* may ensue (f). A final example (g) is that in which a forward and downward lesion affects the motor region controlling tongue movements, producing *dysarthria.*

Since the speech centers are situated in the left cerebral hemisphere in most people, the question arises whether there is any anatomical substratum for hemispheric dominance. For many years it was assumed that the two hemispheres were completely symmetrical. As recently as 1968 two American researchers, Norman Geschwind and Walter Levitsky, actually measured 100 adult brains and found to their surprise that asymmetries can readily be seen. They measured a region known as the *planum temporale,* an extension of Wernicke's area. According to their measurements, that region in the left hemisphere averaged 30 per cent longer than in the right; it was longer in 65 per cent, equal in 24 per cent and smaller in 11 per cent of the brains examined.

Similar asymmetry occurs in the brains of newborn children, suggesting that the anatomical asymmetry associated with language function is present in the human before the onset of language learning and preferred-hand usage. Language localization, to some extent at least, must be present at birth. Even so, some recovery of language function can occur following damage to the language centers, especially in children. The probable explanation is that the right hemisphere is capable of taking over some of the language functions.

Of course, that anatomical method of determining cerebral dominance cannot be used in living subjects. In the 1960s, however, a major breakthrough occurred when a Canadian psychologist, Doreen Kimura, discovered that the *dichotic-listening technique,* which is generally employed in experimental psychology for investigating attention, can be used equally well to investigate cerebral asymmetry.

In dichotic listening, two different words are fed simultaneously into a subject's right and left ears. Kimura noticed that when subjects with known left-hemisphere dominance for language heard series of pairs of digits, the right ear constantly outperformed the left ear. As depicted in Figure 2.4, the reason is that the right ear has a direct connection to the left (language) hemisphere, whereas the left ear's connection is first to the right hemisphere and then via the midline corpus callosum to the left hemisphere.

That finding opened the door to a whole arena of investigations. The left hemisphere, it appears, plays a major role in the decoding of speech, in the analysis of the grammatical structure of sentences, in analytical processing and also in certain nonverbal activities such as the programming of

*Figure 2.4  Basis of the dichotic-listening technique.*

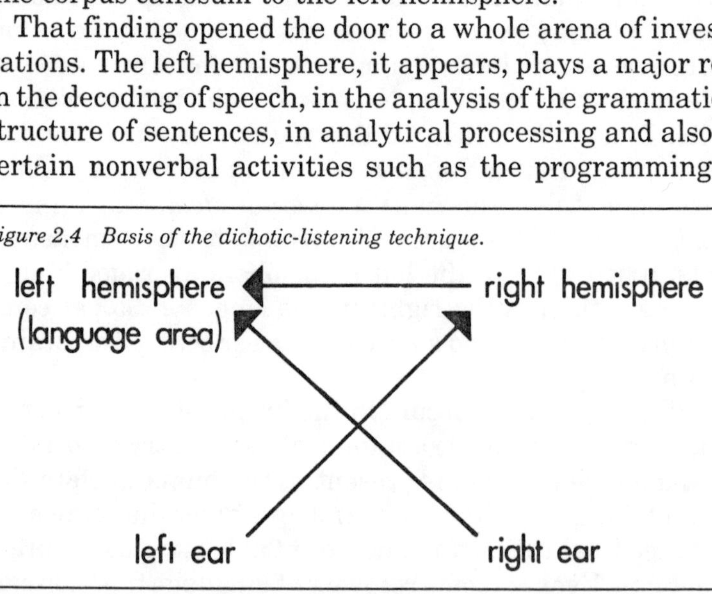

rapid motor sequences, temporal resolution and the control of changes in limb posture. Contemporary studies using dichotic listening reveal, therefore, that the left hemisphere is not exclusively devoted to language functions; Further, the right hemisphere is implicated in some aspects of normal language processing. The degree to which the respective hemispheres contribute to language production appears to vary between individuals and also between languages. For instance, evidence suggests that some languages rely more on left-hemisphere mental abilities than others do.

Signs of the initial stages of development of cerebral dominance are present at birth. The adult level of "language lateralization" is achieved in many children at five years of age. By that age acquisition of a first language is essentially accomplished. Children over five with language deficits do not show an adult level of cerebral dominance.

## Language in Chimpanzees

Why have attempts to teach chimpanzees to speak not been particularly successful? Partly, perhaps, because the larynx and associated structures in chimpanzees are not well suited to human speech. If so, emphasis on the potential *speaking* ability of chimpanzees may actually cloud the issue of their potential *linguistic* ability. Speech itself must be bypassed in order to concentrate on language.

Two American psychologists, Beatrice and Robert Gardner of the University of Nevada, came up with the clever idea of employing a symbolic language such as American sign language (Ameslan). Starting in 1966, the Gardners began to teach Washoe and Lucy, their first chimpanzee pupils, how to converse with them using that gestural language (Fig. 2.5). In the first four years Washoe learned the gestural signs for as many as 200 words—and not just disconnected words, but words strung together by incorporating certain grammatical rules of syntax. Washoe even seems able to construct new words and phrases.

For example, on first seeing a duck landing in a pond,

*Figure 2.5  Two young chimpanzees learning the Ameslan symbol for* listen. *Photograph courtesy of W. B. Lemmon, director of the University of Oklahoma Institute of Primate Studies.*

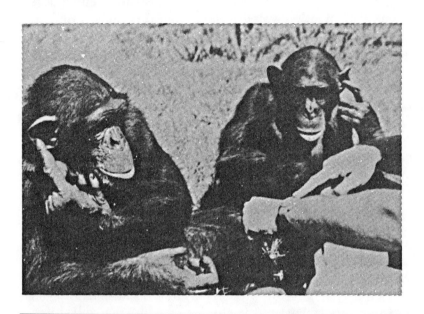

Washoe made the gesture for "water bird." On another occasion she described an orange as an "orange apple." Washoe had never seen an orange before, but recognizing an apple and colors, she devised that creative way of describing an orange. When a small doll was placed on Washoe's cup, the chimp's response was "baby in my drink." Lucy, after some practice, was able to distinguish between the phrases "Roger tickle Lucy" and "Lucy tickle Roger."

Washoe, it appears, has a sense of humor. On one occasion, when riding on her trainer's shoulders, she wet him; her reaction to that was "funny, funny." In a more serious mood she sometimes reads a magazine like a young child, turning over one page after another. Significantly, whenever she recognizes a picture she gestures the appropriate sign.

Another chimpanzee celebrity is Sarah, trained by University of Pennsylvania psychologist David Premack to communicate by means of plastic symbols. She can produce simple sentences like "gimme tickle gimme," but has also learned to understand complex sentences. An example of such a sentence is "If red on green then Sarah take red." She can also understand compound sentences such as "Sarah insert banana in pail, apple in dish."

Particularly impressive was Sarah's accomplishment in actually elaborating for herself the rule for using plurals. Having taught her that "is + pl = are," Premack and his colleagues found that Sarah could not only understand that equation but could also recognize a subject as plural.

Duane Rumbaugh and Susan Savage-Rumbaugh taught chimpanzees to communicate with each other in "Yerkish," an artificial language produced by pressing keys on a console. Francine Patterson claims to have taught a female gorilla over four hundred signs, which were used as insults, rhymes and metaphors.

When we try to go beyond this point, complexities and differences in interpretation arise. Some research workers make more sweeping claims than others about similarities between human and chimpanzee languages. Many claims made in the popular media for the rather exclusive group of linguistic chimpanzees far exceed the evidence. Carl Sagan, in a popular book on the brain *The Dragons of Eden,* waxes eloquent about the intelligence of chimpanzees and about ethical considerations humans should show them in the light of their intelligence. He goes so far as to speculate about the culture and oral traditions that chimpanzees might develop after a few hundred or thousand years of communal use of a complex gestural language. Reminiscent of Pierre Boullé's novel *Monkey Planet* and the less profound *Planet of the Apes,* such speculation bears little relation to scientific reality.

Much less extravagant claims are made by some of the principal research workers. David Premack contends that although apes do not compose sentences of human complexity, neither do they merely memorize words and sentences. Instead, he argues, they display linguistic creativity in composing sentences they have never previously used. In so doing they are inducing a *syntax*. In spite of such linguistic creativity, however, they do not show linguistic novelty, because they cannot change the structure of sentences. Their speech thus shows many similarities to that of the young child. The major difference is that whereas a child is on its way toward adult syntax, the chimpanzee appears to be going no further.

According to Premack, his chimpanzees possess representational capacity in their ability to judge what plastic "words" stand for and to compare two linguistic items. Faced with such a linguistic repertoire, one is tempted to follow popular writers in making broad claims for chimpanzees' supposed humanoid achievements. Yet caution is necessary. Two couples, the Kelloggs and later the Hayeses, spent many years trying to cajole chimps into learning a human language. In the 1940s and '50s Cathy and Keith Hayes spent six years trying to teach Viki to talk, but Viki never got beyond "mamma," "papa," "up" and "cup." Moreover, there can be no doubt that apes are far more adept at learning visual-manual communication than the auditory-vocal processes typical of humans. Hence, no matter how linguistically able chimpanzees may turn out to be, their training in linguistics must be unlike that used for children.

A helpful approach for comparing chimpanzee and human linguistic traits is to compare the linguistic performance of trained chimpanzees with that of two-or three-year-old children. There is little difference in vocabulary size between some of the trained adult chimpanzees and many two-year-old children, so vocabulary alone is not a limitation on chimpanzees' linguistic capacity. When we turn to syntax, however, a different situation holds. As far as present experiments have gone, no chimpanzee has anything resembling the language structure of a normal three-year-old. Although virtually all children use hierarchically structured complex sentences by the beginning of their fourth year, that is not true of the apes.

There is no doubt that some of the chimpanzees, particularly Sarah, have achieved considerable proficiency in using arbitrary symbols to communicate; they are capable of some degree of structural analysis; they can learn a fairly sophisticated substitution technique; and they can use words to describe new types of objects. Premack argues that they can actually generate new words. Others disagree and stress that their inability to do so reflects a basic qualitative difference between human and chimpanzee use of language.

A voice of dissent in this debate is that of Columbia University psychologist, Herbert Terrace. Working with an infant chimpanzee, Nim (short for Neam Chimpsky), Terrace found that after forty-four months of intensive sign-language drill Nim failed to master either the rudiments of grammar or sentence construction. Nim's language showed little spontaneity. On examining video tapes of Nim and other chimpanzees, Terrace concluded that chimpanzees' utterances are imitations of their teachers' unintentional clues and gestures, and rotelike repetitions of memorized combinations. In Terrace's words: "Apes can learn many isolated symbols (as can dogs, horses, and other non-human species), but they show no unequivocal evidence of mastering the conversational, semantic, or syntactic organization of language."

Whatever one's position in the debate, the dissimilarities between the language of an ape and a normal three-year-old child are striking. We are left with a fundamental question: Why don't apes use human language? However remarkable their linguistic achievements, they are far from the human use of human language. The experimental successes clearly highlight their limitations.

Several responses have been made to the question posed. An immediate possibility is a deficient chimpanzee vocal tract, which may be incapable of producing the full range of speech sounds. Psychologist John Limber has argued that "the (non-human) primates could not produce human speech even if they had something to say." Yet that cannot be the sole explanation. After all, there are cases of humans with exceedingly severe deformations of their vocal tracts managing to produce intelligible speech. To quote Limber again: "Engaging in this complex activity not only requires having something to say but also the specific rules for encoding that intention and a vocal apparatus for generating the appropriate signal."

The next level of explanation is a neuroanatomical one. Human and chimpanzee brains differ in organization of the language centers. The anatomical differences probably contribute to the linguistic differences. In particular, the angular gyrus (Fig. 2.1) is better developed in the human brain than in the chimpanzee's. That is the region that enables human language to be used to refer to objects independent of emotional considerations, opening the way to elaboration of rational thought. Also, the asymmetry of the brain in the temporal-lobe language region is present in the chimpanzee brain to a lesser extent than in the human.

Perhaps, in the end, human language has a genetic base and is more or less independent of intelligence. If that is so, children are genetically predisposed to learn one of the many human languages, but chimpanzees are not. Linguist Noam Chomsky claims that children have within them an innate, universal system of syntax which makes them competent to understand and generate speech. Rules of grammar, according to his postulate, operate independently of meaning. That plausible-sounding explanation smacks of being too inclusive; it may simply be a last stop when all other explanations have been found wanting. Even so, there must be basic organizational differences between human and chimpanzee brains to account for the cognitive and linguistic differences, although so far they have largely eluded neuroscientists.

## The Human Brain and Humanness

The question, "Why don't apes use human language?" inevitably raises another, "Why are apes and humans different?" What is it about their brains that distinguishes human beings from chimpanzees? It may be objected that to phrase the dilemma in such terms is misleading, yet this is the point to which discussion of the linguistic potential and limitations of chimpanzees has brought us.

Human beings, in their thinking, can make and use abstract concepts which, in turn, open the way to the invention of new ideas and to the interplay of ideas. The latter attribute calls forth imagination, from which arise poetic language and scientific concepts. For concept formation to be adequately utilized, however, another trait is essential. That trait is generalization, which lies at the heart of all human systems of explanation and forecasting. Being capable of thinking in abstract and general terms, humans are in a position to attempt to understand themselves and their world. When one looks at oneself as a person and as an individual, *self-knowledge* and *self-consciousness* begin to be evident.

Because they possess a degree of self-knowledge, individuals are continually confronted by a demand not only to know but to understand themselves as human beings. Integral to that understanding is an awareness of other people and thus a comparison of how the individual matches up to others. One result of encounters with other people and their images is a growing awareness of "who I am" as a person. Such an awareness constitutes self-consciousness, which carries with it the implication that self-conscious creatures *know that they know.* Self-knowledge of that kind has traditionally been regarded as a uniquely human capacity, although some commentators on chimpanzees' efforts at mastery of language claim that chimps, too, demonstrate such capacity. (The humility of that claim is matched only by its wishful thinking!) Self-consciousness insures that human beings continually ask questions about themselves, their existence, their destiny and about any and every aspect of the world. Surely chimpanzees have never begun to formulate, let alone think through, those sorts of questions.

Human conceptual attributes lead to the creation of new ideas, to the imagining of new solutions to old problems, and to questioning of one's own existence. In other words, those attributes have bestowed creativity and inventiveness on mankind, so that human beings are in the unique position of being able to "create their own world." They can devise new strategies for existence; they can look to the future, knowing they are intimately involved in what form it will take. That is human culture, dependent in a fundamental sense on our ability to communicate linguistically, to create and to ask questions.

Our human capacity for molding our external environment is, however, just one facet of our intellectual attributes. The complementary facet is that each of us as an individual being is characterized by a desire to know and to be known. Each of us has a sense of our own personal uniqueness and transience, so that one day we know we will cease to be. Our self-awareness is closely allied with our *death-awareness*. Life is therefore a search for meaning, as we attempt to discover who we are and whether there is a rationale for our being and even for the existence of the universe itself. We are closely related to the universe, even though we fear its immensity and intransigence.

The finiteness of human life goads human existence. Individuals are transient and insignificant, however immense the scope of some human intellectual endeavors. Knowing so much about ourselves as biological and social beings, we know we will die and, in the absence of a world view incorporating spiritual as well as biological considerations, we face anxiety and uncertainty. Death-awareness is a prelude to what Theodosius Dobzhansky has described as man's ultimate concern, that is, his concern with things beyond himself and his present life; it is concern with the infinite. Man must make sense of who he is; he cannot get away from his quest for meaning in life. That quest appears to be an essential aspect of the human biological makeup.

Not surprisingly, therefore, man's life is dominated by a search for truth and characterized by a concern for moral values. Individuals may profess no interest in those pursuits but the human race has been unable to escape from them. They remind us that human dimensions include nonbiological obligations, rooted in our relationship to, and awareness of, God. Religious dimensions appear integral to our biological makeup; that is, a yearning for what is beyond us reflects a deeply felt human need.

In our full human dimensions, we are rooted in nature but we are also formed in the image of God. We contend with the vagaries of the physical cosmos, but we also have to meet God's standards and demands. We come face to face with biological and social forces, but we will also come face to face with One who is superior to us and to whom we must ultimately answer: God. Capable of a level of religious experience and spiritual existence quite different from all other living things, we are created to respond to God's gracious Word in personal love and trust. Indeed, only in such response can we fulfill the potential of *being* complete human beings.

What does it mean to *be* human and to *act* in a human fashion? Humanness includes an awareness of oneself as an individual, something of which chimpanzees may be capable as they recognize their images in a mirror. But it also includes an understanding of oneself and of one's goals, implicit within which is an ability to judge oneself, one's description of the world and one's goals. Human beings make moral and aesthetic judgments. We are self-reflective beings. Our self-reflection begins to manifest itself early in childhood when we make judgments about, for instance, the correctness of sentences being used. At present it is impossible to know if any aspects of such self-reflection are shared by apes, but it is clear that self-reflection demands far more than mere ability to ask questions, describe states of affairs and make truth claims.

Humanness demands creativity, the ability to think and act in totally new ways, to imagine new solutions and see things in novel forms. Creativity means that human beings can change themselves; they can adapt themselves and their environment to meet new demands. They can transform almost everything they touch. Creativity of that order, unknown among nonhumans, is dependent on a level of intelligence found only within the genus *Homo*. Richard Leakey and Roger Lewin in their book *Origins* state: "The secret of the human mind is that rather than having the ability to learn variants of *specific* tasks or behavior patterns, it simply has the *ability to* learn, to be adaptive to practically anything that the environment has to offer."

Also implicit within humanness is a potential for responding to the overtures of God. Individuals may not respond at all, or their response may vary from warm anticipation to outright hostility. Nevertheless, all our responses signify an interaction with God, something uniquely human.

What then does it mean to be human? On the one hand, being human implies a brain capable of integrating signals received from the outside world, learning from them and communicating with others of its kind, so that together a whole community can learn and increase in wisdom. Such a brain must have a large cerebral cortex, well-developed and intimately interrelated tertiary association areas (chapter 3) and, therefore, greatly expanded parietal and temporal lobes. Specialized language centers must be closely integrated with special sensory systems. On the other hand, being human means originating from God's purposes and achieving both significance and freedom within God's designs. Such beings are free to go their own way, but the freedom that will enhance their human status is grounded within, and developed according to, the precepts of their Creator.

Supremely, perhaps, humanness implies a knowledge of death, with all that flows from such knowledge. Would it be possible to impart to an ape the knowledge that it will die?

If so, would an ape appreciate the significance of that knowledge for its present existence? In other words, would that knowledge modify the way in which it now lives? Those questions touch on a fundamental element in the gap separating apes and human beings. Critical as language is to humanness, it is a vehicle for more profound elements of what *being human* means. Unless it can be shown that the linguistic capacities of chimpanzees can serve as harbingers of an awareness of transience, the distinction between human and nonhuman primates will remain unblurred.

## Two Hemispheres in One Brain

A conundrum remaining from a foregoing discussion is how, with two such different cerebral hemispheres, human beings can be blissfully unaware of an appalling chasm in their personalities. It may not be too fanciful to suggest that, potentially at least, each of us has within our skull two brains which, under normal circumstances, somehow manage to function as a smoothly integrated whole.

As long ago as 1844, A. L. Wigan, in a book entitled *The Duality of the Mind,* was proposing that possession of two hemispheres might well mean the existence of two minds within one person. Wigan was led to that startling possibility by a post-mortem examination of an apparently healthy individual who, it emerged, had only one cerebral hemisphere. From that discovery, Wigan concluded that, if only one hemisphere is required to have a mind or to be a person, two functioning hemispheres may presage two minds. If so, those two minds may come into conflict from time to time.

Wigan's ideas, which were many years ahead of their time, attracted no notice because little was known about the interrelationship of the two hemispheres and because consciousness was then a subject of metaphysics rather than neuroscience. Interest in such ideas had to await experimental investigations on the seemingly unproductive problem of the functions of the corpus callosum.

As described in the first chapter, the two cerebral hemispheres are normally joined together across the midline by a bundle of fibers known as the corpus callosum (Fig. 1.10). That structure is one of the so-called *commissures,* or bundles of fibers linking equivalent centers or areas on the two sides of the brain. Other important commissures are the anterior and hippocampal commissures.

An amazing feature of the corpus callosum deceived investigators for many years: cutting it did not seem to affect the experimental animal or human patient. Indeed, a distinguished experimental psychologist is said to have remarked half-seriously in the early 1950s that the corpus callosum's role is "to keep the hemispheres from sagging." His statement was based in large measure on the studies of A. J. Akelaitis on twenty-six patients whose corpus callosum and anterior commissure had been completely or partially cut in an attempt to keep severe epileptic seizures from spreading from one hemisphere to the other. Akelaitis's assessment of those patients led him to conclude that the operation was remarkably successful, alleviating the epileptic seizures and leaving the patients apparently normal in every way.

The corpus callosum was thus an enigma for neurologists. After all, it contains 200 million nerve fibers, representing approximately 2 per cent of the total number of nerve cells in the cortex. Thus, it was difficult to believe that the corpus callosum had no function.

The first experiments on the "split brain" were carried out in the cat by Ronald Myers and Roger Sperry at the University of Chicago. Myers found that, when the optic chiasm (the place where optic fibers running from the eyes to the brain cross from one side of the head to the other) is severed, information presented to one eye and hence one hemisphere is still able to cross to the other hemisphere (Fig. 2.6). In other words, transfer of information between the two hemispheres must be using a route other than the optic chiasm, the most likely candidate being the corpus callosum. That hypothesis led to the first "split-brain" investigation, in

*Figure 2.6  Overview of the brain of a cat or monkey depicting the corpus callosum and optic tracts. Both carry fibers from one side of the brain to the other and have been cut in this "split brain."*

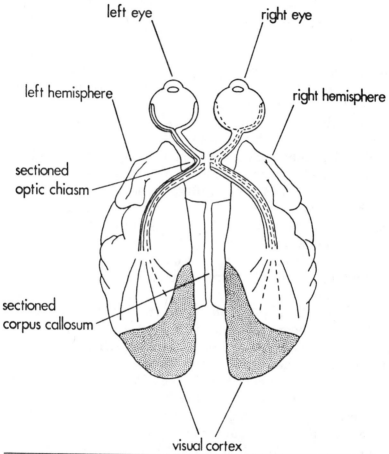

left eye                    right eye

left hemisphere                    right hemisphere

sectioned
optic chiasm

sectioned
corpus callosum

visual cortex

which both the optic chiasm and corpus callosum are split in the midline. Beginning in the early 1950s, Sperry and his associates were responsible for many series of such experiments in cats and monkeys, laying a basis for subsequent human operations. Let us first consider some of those pioneering animal investigations.

Cats and monkeys with split brains show no obvious disturbances of coordination; they maintain their internal functions and perform as well as control animals in standard tests of learning ability. What is more, there is no change in their personality or temperament. When a split-brain animal is tested for performance of the two halves of the brain separately, however, an important principle emerges: *that which is experienced or learned by one cerebral hemisphere cannot be transferred to the other one.* Although that restriction has few consequences for the ordinary course of life for such animals, it does lead to some bizarre disabilities.

Since each hemisphere of a split-brain animal is operating as an independent unit, it will respond as an independent unit. For one hemisphere to learn a particular solution to a problem does not in any way influence the other hemisphere, which is capable of learning a diametrically opposite solution to the same problem. The split-brain animal acts as though it has two entirely separate brains. Perhaps animals with two cerebral hemispheres do possess two brains, at least under abnormal circumstances. The problem is enormously subtle.

Once the general principles of separating the two sides of the brain had been elaborated in animal studies, equivalent operations could be undertaken in humans. The reason for such operations has usually been intractable epilepsy. From the 1960s onward, about twenty such operations have been carried out and analyzed. Many have been performed in California by Joseph Bogen. In the operation the fibers of the corpus callosum and anterior commissure are sectioned.

Consider the example of a right-handed person, with a dominant left cerebral hemisphere and, therefore, with the speech centers in that left hemisphere (Fig. 2.7). After the operation, most activities involving the left cerebral hemisphere and the right side of the body are performed in a perfectly adequate manner. The patient can read anything presented to his right visual field (which is projected to his left hemisphere); he can recognize and name objects in his right visual field, and he can execute commands to move his right

*Figure 2.7 Overview of the human brain illustrating the two cerebral hemispheres, some of the operations localized in each hemisphere, and the way in which each visual field is represented in the opposite hemisphere. The corpus callosum (sectioned) and optic tracts are shown but are not labeled.*

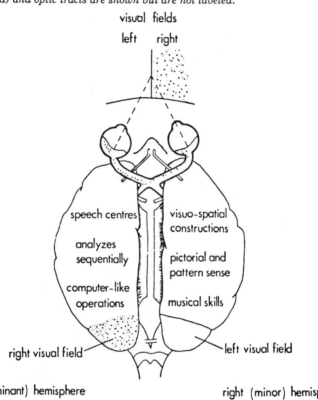

hand, right foot, or any part of the right side of his body.

But things are not so clear-cut on the left side of the body. The patient is unable to read anything in his left visual field, and he cannot write *at all* with his left hand. Further, he is incapable of carrying out verbal commands requiring movement of his left hand or leg.

The reason for this odd behavior is that the *speech areas,* located in the dominant left hemisphere, are no longer connected to the right hemisphere which is responsible for the

actions of the left side of the body. Cutting the corpus callosum, therefore, means that the right hemisphere is unable
to direct the left hand to do things connected with speech,
which includes writing. Also, when an object is presented
in the left field of vision (projecting to his right hemisphere),
the patient can see it but can neither explain it nor write
about it. Similarly, he can see a printed page in his left field
of vision but is unable to understand it because there is no
communication between the right and left hemispheres.
This type of patient, therefore, is displaying effects known as
"word-blindness" and "word-deafness," both of which result

*Figure 2.8 Arrangement used for testing symptoms produced by sectioning the
corpus callosum in a human being. Courtesy of R. W. Sperry and the Association
for Research in Nervous and Mental Disease, Inc.*

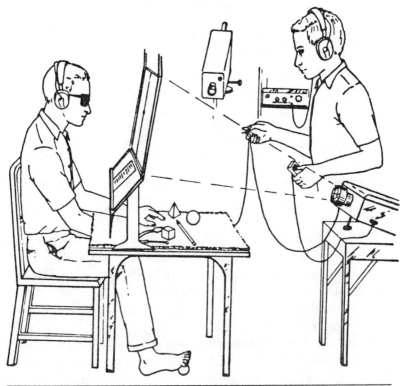

from faulty communication between the two hemispheres.

The experimental arrangement for testing symptoms produced by commissural section is shown in Figure 2.8. The subject fixes his gaze on a central spot on the screen, after which a word is flashed for one-tenth of a second on either the left or right side of the screen. Behind the screen are placed various objects which can be handled by the subject's hands but which are hidden from his view. In that way it is

*Figure 2.9  Arrangement for demonstrating that a word projected to the right hemisphere of a split-brain patient can be understood and acted upon. Courtesy of R. W. Sperry and the Association for Research in Nervous and Mental Disease, Inc.*

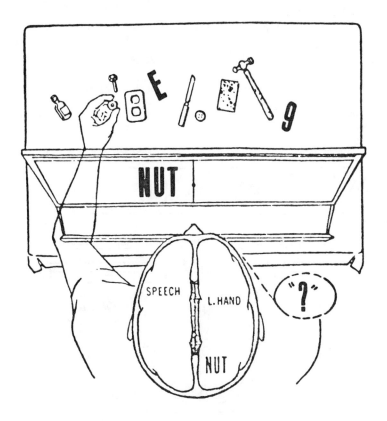

possible to test the two sides of a patient's split brain separately (Fig. 2.7).

If the word *nut* is flashed on the left side of the screen (Fig. 2.9), it is picked up by the right hemisphere which programs the left hand. The subject, having seen that word, is able to use his left hand to find a nut among the array of objects hidden from view behind the screen. That demonstrates that the right hemisphere displays an intelligent understanding of common names and can program the left hand to find common objects. If the subject is questioned about what he is doing, however, he is at a total loss. The subject, as a speaking individual, is completely ignorant of the whole operation. In other words, to follow Sperry's line of reasoning, the goings-on in the right hemisphere are unknown to the speaking subject who is in liaison only with the goings-on in the left hemisphere with its speech centers.

---

*Figure 2.10   In this experimental setup, only the word* BAND, *picked up by the left hemisphere, enters the split-brain subject's consciousness and is verbally reported. Courtesy of R. W. Sperry and the Association for Research and Mental Disease, Inc.*

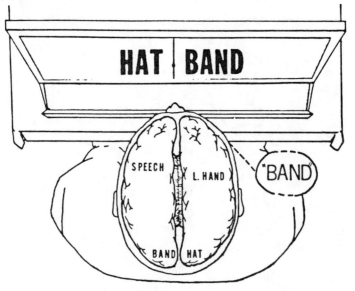

A clear illustration of the cleavage is provided by the test shown in Figure 2.10. In this instance, the word *hatband* is flashed on the screen, *hat* being to the left of the central spot and *band* to the right. The word *hat* is picked up by the right hemisphere and *band* by the left hemisphere. As the latter is the speaking hemisphere, the subject is aware of *band* but has no idea of the existence of *hat*. Consequently, when asked what type of band the test is about, the subject guesses at random. Clearly, a person with a split brain is conscious of information in his speaking left hemisphere, but is unaware of information being acquired by his non-speaking right hemisphere.

We must beware of oversimplification. The right hemisphere, even when it is the minor or nonspeaking one, has some linguistic capabilities. That can be demonstrated by an adaptation of the previous experiments so that a few words are displayed on the screen for a period of time which is long enough for them to be seen by both eyes and thus fed into both hemispheres. Then one of those words, *book,* for example, is flashed on the left side of the screen. The subject is instructed to write the word down using his left hand. The remarkable feature of this experiment is that he is able to do so, although only the right hemisphere is implicated in recognizing the word and subsequently in controlling the left hand. Even more remarkable is that the subject does not know what he has written, because the script is concealed from his view and, of course, the left hemisphere with its speech centers has played no role in the whole process. He knows from the motion of his hand that he has written something but, because he cannot see it and because information is not being transferred from his right to left hemispheres, he illustrates once again an ignorance of events going on within and controlled by his nonspeaking hemisphere.

Not only can the right hemisphere direct the left hand to write simple words, but it is quite competent at reproducing three-dimensional models even though it has to work via the

*Figure 2.11  The left hand (controlled by the right cerebral hemisphere) is more competent at simple geometric representations than is the right hand (controlled by the left hemisphere).*

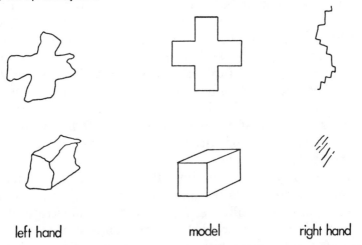

| left hand | model | right hand |

inexperienced left hand. From Figure 2.11 it can also be deduced that the right hand and its controlling left hemisphere are surprisingly incompetent at simple geometric representations. The right hand's copy of such a design preserves the *elements* of it but loses the *essence* of its form.

The difference between the two hemispheres can be summed up by saying that the difference is more of style than of content. The left hemisphere emphasizes logical precision and exact categorization, whereas the right is more concerned with wholeness or, as a psychologist might say, with the formation of a "Gestalt" (pattern, configuration).

## Respective Functions of the Hemispheres

The foregoing experimental evidence on split-brain subjects has provided distinct clues about the respective functions of the left and right hemispheres. These clues, coupled with many other psychological tests, enable us to construct rough lists of the hemispheres' abilities. One such list is shown in Figure 2.12. The left hemisphere, which is usually

*Figure 2.12    Respective functions of the two cerebral hemispheres.*

## CEREBRAL  HEMISPHERES

| LEFT | RIGHT |
|---|---|
| speech (verbal) | largely non–verbal |
| fine imaginative details | sequential operations |
| arithmetical | geometrical / spatial |
| digital computer-like | analog computer-like |
| analytical | holistic / synthetic |
| sequential | pictorial / pattern sense |
| ideational | musical / poetical |

the dominant one, is the verbal one; it can make itself felt because the subject is aware of its information store. In addition it is specialized to deal with fine imaginative details, so that it sorts out information in an analytical and sequential fashion. It also has arithmetical-like characteristics, and is sometimes compared to a digital computer. The right or minor hemisphere, by contrast, is largely nonverbal. Its assets are that it processes information simultaneously; it is rather like an analog computer building up whole pictures and discerning patterns rather than details. It is superior to the left hemisphere in all kinds of geometrical and perspective drawings, its goal appearing to be the establishment of holistic images and the synthesis of information. These ideas are strengthened by its involvement in musical appreciation, which is coherent and synthetic, depending on a sequential input of sounds. It may be that poetry is also a right-hemisphere function.

Enormous interest has been created by these findings, leading to discussions of what might happen if conflict occurs between a person's two hemispheres, the extent to which Western thought relies on left-hemisphere functions and Eastern thought on right-hemisphere ones, and the implications for education of having to teach children with differing left- and right-hemisphere abilities. In some quarters the respective functions of the hemispheres have been so overaccentuated that the functional differences between the hemispheres have come to imply their specialization. With the further assumption that the functions of the two hemispheres are incompatible, the brain is pictured as a battleground of warring factions. Viewing brain function in that framework makes it extremely difficult to gain any feeling for the brain as an integrated whole. So we must ask whether a two-brain model is misleading.

The issue is quite complex. On the one hand, there can be no doubt about the enhanced ability of the left hemisphere for an analytical mode of working and of the right hemisphere for a coherent one. On the other, each hemisphere often has a hint of the attributes of its opposite. For instance, although the right hemisphere has a relative advantage over the left one on some perceptual tests, perceptual processing is possible in both half-brains.

Michael Gazzaniga argues that distinctions between the two hemispheres arising from split-brain studies are exaggerated, because the superiority of the right hemisphere over the left on a variety of tasks is a consequence of the inclusion of manipulative and spatial activities in the experimental design of the tests. It is clear that the left hemisphere is minimally involved in manipulative and spatial functions. The reason, according to Gazzaniga, is that the two functions of language and manipulo-spatiality compete for space in the brain. During early childhood, language emerges first, generally becoming located in the left hemisphere, thereby relegating the later-developing manipulo-spatiality to an equivalent region of the right hemisphere.

Gazzaniga's speculative idea is interesting in that it views the brain as an integrated whole. Although some functions are better developed in one hemisphere than the other, there is no opposition between them. Should the appearance of a particular function be delayed during an individual's development, it may be able to establish itself later on in the opposite hemisphere. Accordingly, the cerebral hemispheres in humans work together to maintain the integrity of mental functioning, and hence the wholeness of the person. That, I believe, is an important principle which should not be forgotten during discussion of the respective functions of the two hemispheres.

Up to this point the models used for comparing the right and left hemispheres have been pathological ones. Fascinating as split brains are, they represent an abnormal brain. What we now need to ask is whether normal people doing ordinary, everyday things make use of the lateral specialization of the brain. If so, what is the nature of such specialization in ordinary people?

Such questions were posed by psychologists Robert Ornstein and David Galin at the Langley-Porter Neuropsychiatric Institute in San Francisco. Using electroencephalograms (EEGs) they found that, in a normal subject, the right hemisphere "idled" during writing and the left hemisphere when arranging blocks. Extending their study to other subjects and using a greater variety of tests, they came to the conclusion that there is a greater left-hemisphere activity in verbal tasks and greater right-hemisphere activity in spatial tasks. From that baseline, they sought to differentiate between occasions on which a person uses the left hemisphere and occasions on which the right one is used. It might even be, they reasoned, that certain individuals utilize one hemisphere more than the other; some people might rely more on their left hemisphere with its verbal-analytic mode, others on their right hemisphere with its spatial-holistic approach.

In order to test that hypothesis, two groups of people were selected: lawyers as representatives of left-hemisphere-dependent people and sculptors as representatives of those primarily dependent on the right hemisphere. Although a consistent difference between left- and right-hemisphere activity in verbal and spatial processing was again obtained, marked right/left differences between the lawyers and sculptors did not appear. Notwithstanding that setback, Ornstein and Galin noted that, when the activity within each hemisphere was examined, the lawyers showed consistently greater changes in left-hemisphere activity on all tasks given them. They concluded that lawyers differ from sculptors mainly in the use of their left hemisphere.

Interesting as that conclusion is, it would be unwise to place too much stress on alleged differences. Differences do appear to exist between right- and left-hemisphere capabilities and also in the extent to which different individuals depend on one or other of the hemispheres. In the final analysis, however, the exigencies of normal living demand that both hemispheres be utilized; an integrated life depends on an integrated brain. Certainly we differ as individuals because our brains differ. Major personality differences may reflect a predominance under certain circumstances of one hemisphere. It would be unwise, however, to extrapolate from those concepts to the concept of right-hemisphere individuals or of right-hemisphere professions, or the converse.

## Significance of Two Hemispheres
A discussion such as the preceding one confronts us with an

exceedingly perplexing question: Why are two hemispheres necessary? Although no fully convincing answer can be given, one can at least attempt an analysis of the *significance* of two hemispheres.

The unlikely starting point for such a discussion is the observation that individuals can exist with only *one* hemisphere. Several case histories of the removal of a cerebral hemisphere (hemispherectomy) are available for study and are remarkable in what they reveal. As one would anticipate in light of the functions of the hemispheres, the consequences differ greatly depending on which hemisphere is removed.

Excision of the minor hemisphere under local anesthesia results in symptoms that, except for paralysis of the opposite side of the body, are essentially the same as those following split-brain operations. There is no loss of the patient's consciousness or self-awareness. Not surprisingly, removal of the dominant hemisphere carries with it much more serious consequences, including almost complete aphasia. In spite of that, some residual consciousness remains and there may be some recovery of primitive linguistic functions.

These descriptions apply to adults. By contrast, in infants up to five years of age, the functions of the dominant hemisphere can be effectively transferred to its minor counterpart. Consequently, removal of the left dominant hemisphere during the first few years of life does not have the catastrophic consequences for language development of later removal of that hemisphere. Speech is transferred to the minor hemisphere which thus assumes the role of the talking hemisphere, but with some losses of neural functioning. Complete transfer of language functions, as occurs in excision of the dominant hemisphere in infancy, leads to a deterioration of some of the nonlinguistic functions of the one remaining hemisphere. It seems, therefore, that one hemisphere cannot accommodate the range of functions normally found within the two hemispheres together. Hence two hemispheres appear to be necessary for no more profound reason than that of providing sufficient "room" for normal hemisphere functions.

That conclusion fails to account for the principles governing distribution of functions between the hemispheres. A possible contribution to that distribution has already been mentioned: preference seems to be given to the language centers, which develop early, with nonlinguistic functions fitting around the language centers. Although more investigation is required to clarify that possibility, there can be no escape from the significance of the language centers. Their role in the human cerebral hemispheres clearly impinges on the meaning of humanness.

What makes human beings human has been shown earlier to include conscious awareness by the individual. From the split-brain studies we know that the left hemisphere has conscious awareness of the external world. But what about the right hemisphere? This is where difficulties arise and where neurobiology takes on distinct philosophical overtones.

For Roger Sperry, the minor right hemisphere has a conscious system of its own, and both hemispheres may be conscious simultaneously in different, even mutually conflicting, mental experiences that run in parallel. If the right hemisphere does have a consciousness of its own, its existence is normally obscured by its lack of a linguistic means of expressing itself. A similar position was arrived at by Michael Gazzaniga after study of one of his split-brain subjects. A corollary of this view is that the mechanisms of human consciousness can be split along with the splitting of the brain, so that a split-brain patient may demonstrate double consciousness.

Sir John Eccles, however, questions the validity of a double-consciousness interpretation even in split-brain subjects. It is his contention that, because we lack linguistic communication with the minor right hemisphere, it is not feasible to test for the existence within it of any consciously experiencing being. For Eccles, the dominant left hemisphere is the only part of the brain in direct liaison with the conscious self or the self-conscious mind and, consequently, is the only part of the brain under the control of the latter. For Eccles that conclusion has far-reaching philosophical connotations; it serves as the basis for an "interactionist" model of the relationship between mind and brain. We shall return to that topic in the final chapter.

It is easy to speak about the two hemispheres acting in conflict and to imagine bizarre scenarios. Not even a vestige of credibility can be assigned to those possibilities, however, until the role of the hemispheres has been placed in the context of brain function as a whole. Far more research on hemisphere functions in the normal brain must precede any acceptance of double consciousness and conflicting cerebral hemispheres as a reality.

Nevertheless, greater awareness of the heterogeneity of mental ability may have far-reaching repercussions for the development of mental skills. As long ago as the thirteenth century, Roger Bacon distinguished between two modes of knowing: argument and experience. Perhaps it would be simplistic to relate one of these to the left hemisphere and the other to the right. Yet the contrasts are instructive and may provide clues to learning—which educators should not lightly dismiss. Such ideas in alliance with the brain-consciousness paradigm substantiate the necessity of a *whole* brain for a unitary appreciation of and response to the world. Without a whole brain even the simplest tasks become quixotic and the subtleties of normal existence assume gigantic proportions.

Whole persons are as important as functioning brains. People, whatever their strong or weak points, need to be accepted for what they are. Every individual, and every group of individuals, has a potentially important contribution to make to the human family. In no sense can it be said that right-hemisphere-dependent individuals (if there are such people) are superior to left-hemisphere-dependent ones or vice versa. Judgments of that nature are subjective, reflecting only the biases of the one making the judgment. Such comparisons deny the oneness of the human race in the image of God. Different groups, reflecting different personality traits and perhaps different hemisphere characteristics, contribute to different extents to the predominant cultures of our time. What is required is that we appreciate the contributions of these diversities, rather than elevate one type at the expense of others.

People are people, and all are made in the image and likeness of God. All people are of concern to God, whose relationship to mankind is person-centered rather than ability-centered. That feature of God's character was brought out clearly in the life of Jesus, whose great concern was for the downtrodden of society: the sick, the dispossessed, the forsaken, the sinners. On such persons he bestowed the utmost compassion, whereas for the arrogant and self-righteous he reserved his severest strictures and most critical rebukes.

It is in that light that we need to view the differential hemisphere characteristics. There is no point in trying to hide differences that exist among human beings. All do not possess equivalent brains or equivalent abilities. By virtue of their creation by God and for his purposes, however, all have a dignity bestowed upon them—regardless of left-hemisphere abilities, right-hemisphere abilities or a comparative lack of both. All people should be provided with the opportunities to fulfill themselves to as great an extent as possible. It seems to me that Christians should have such a vision for all people, both individuals and cultural subgroups within society.

# 3

## Damaged Brains and Diseased Personalities

OUR CHIEF CONCERN IN the preceding chapters has been the brain as a healthy functioning unit. Our interest has centered on how the brain as a whole functions and on how some of its component parts work together as the functioning whole we term a normal brain. In the process we have also considered some consequences of isolating one region from another, such as, the right hemisphere from the left.

### Brain and Personality
A healthy brain and a healthy personality are integrally linked, with the brain providing the building-blocks essential for the integrity of the personality. Individuals as we know them derive their unique characteristics from the brains they possess. Damage a man's or a woman's brain, therefore, and you damage their personality and perhaps much that makes them the individuals they are (Fig. 3.1).

Linked to the assumption of an intimate connection be-

Figure 3.1 *Diagrammatic representation of the intimate relationship between the brain and personality of two individuals, A and B. When each of these brains is damaged in some way, the personality of the corresponding individual is modified. The two brains of A, labeled I and II, represent A's brain in youth and old age, linked with the same recognizable personality.*

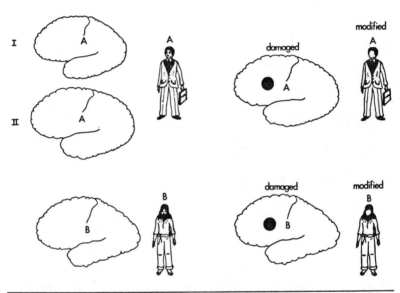

tween an individual's brain and personality is an allied assumption, namely, that what we are as individuals is unchanging. True, we recognize that people grow old, and the aging process is accompanied by readily acknowledged traits: a diminution in the acuteness of memory and a modification of reactions to events and issues. Yet underlying such superficial changes is an apparently unyielding permanence; the elderly remain essentially the same people (Fig. 3.1). What people are in their innermost selves is unchangeable. Since selfhood is continuous, it is generally taken for granted that individuals' personalities are indelible features of all they represent.

In many senses that view is correct. We recognize people after intervals of many years, not simply because their appearance is more or less as we remember them, but because their personalities are much the same. Their outlook on life, their likes and dislikes, their reactions to people and events are at least recognizable. Even if their views have altered, sometimes in major ways, we still see them as the same people we once knew. What gives people their continuity, and what does it mean? Can it be lost?

When we think about such questions we are immediately confronted by two examples of changing personalities. Children grow and develop and learn how to respond to new demands made on them by their environment. Clearly they are changing, their personalities are being molded and transformed by interaction with their environment, until some sort of recognizable stability is attained. At the other end of the scale, elderly persons are undergoing senile changes, with loss of memory, perhaps, fearfulness of anything new and regression into the comforting world of their bygone childhood.

Aging, with the possibility of physical and mental loss, frightens most people. It highlights the fragility of human personality and emphasizes the knife-edge on which we walk as human beings. We are finite creatures, knowing nothing of the inextinguishability of gods. We seem to be dependent on the integrity of our bodies and, supremely, on the integrity of our brains. Hence it behooves us to study at some length what happens to people when their brains are damaged. We shall examine the extent to which personality is dependent on the brain, and also the nature of personality loss following brain injury. That will help clarify the personal responsibility of brain-damaged individuals and society's expectations of their capabilities.

## Case Histories

Three case histories will set the scene for discussion of the interrelationship between brain damage and personality. *Case 1.* Our first case goes back to 13 September 1848, when a twenty-five-year-old construction foreman, Phineas P. Gage, was working on the new line of the Rutland and Burlington Railroad near Cavendish, Vermont. He was in charge of a gang of men about to blast away a rock by pouring gunpowder into a hole drilled in it. The powder accidentally exploded and propelled an iron tamping rod, 3.5 feet long and 1.25 inches in diameter, through Gage's skull (Fig. 3.2). The rod shot through his left cheek, emerged from a hole on the right side of his skull and then landed several yards away on the rocks.

Unbelievably, Phineas Gage was not killed. Within a few minutes of the accident, Gage was conscious and was asking his stunned workmates about the whereabouts of his rod. After being taken by ox cart to the Cavendish Hotel, Gage stepped off the cart and walked up a long flight of stairs to have his profusely bleeding wounds dressed. The local physician, John M. Harlow, could hardly believe his eyes, especially when he found he could insert his fingers into the holes in Gage's skull. Even more convinced of Gage's imminent demise was the local cabinetmaker, who immediately set to work on a coffin.

Phineas Gage was not to be kept out of the record books that easily, however. Although for a few days he was seriously ill from infected wounds and loss of blood, he eventually recovered. By mid-November he was wandering around Cavendish, ready for the new life before him. His recovery was no more dramatic than his new life: in many respects, Gage was a new person. Before the accident he had been soft-

*Figure 3.2   Photograph of the tamping bar which was driven through the skull of Phineas Gage. Courtesy of the Warren Anatomical Museum, Harvard Medical School, Boston.*

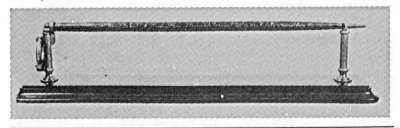

spoken, purposeful, capable and efficient; after the accident he became bombastic, with little evidence of purpose in his existence and with a violent temper. In a paper published in 1868, John Harlow, commenting on these personality changes, wrote: "He is fitful, irreverent, indulging at times in the grossest profanity (which was not previously his custom), manifesting but little deference for his fellows ... at times pertinaciously obstinate, yet capricious and vacillating, devising many plans of future operation, which are no sooner arranged than they are abandoned." Harlow quoted Gage's friends to the effect that he was "no longer Gage."

Rejected by the railroad company and plagued by an aimless wanderlust, Gage became a fairground attraction, drifting around North and South America exhibiting himself and the tamping bar. He ended up in San Francisco, where he died in 1860—a sad end for such an important, though unintentional, scientific experiment.

Phineas Gage was a living monument to the fact that personality can be dramatically transformed by destroying part of the brain, in his case the frontal lobes (Fig. 1.12) and their connections with the remainder of the brain. He was a forerunner of the intentionally applied destruction of equivalent frontal lobe tissue in the classical frontal leucotomy operations of the 1940s and '50s (chapter 4). It is ironic that a procedure that ruined the life of one man should be used therapeutically a century later in thousands of others, although additional considerations came into play in the therapeutic realm. The destruction of frontal lobe tissue in Gage's brain proved cataclysmic for him. We can surmise that, in his pre-accident days, he would have opted for a life of obscure fulfillment rather than his post-accident notoriety and dubious honor of having his skull displayed in the Harvard Medical School museum (Fig. 3.3). It is even more intriguing to wonder what the post-accident, "model-two" Phineas Gage thought. That raises immense questions to which we shall return in the final section of this chapter.

*Case 2.* In 1953 another accident occurred—this time a

*Figure 3.3 Phineas Gage's skull and life mask. The skull shows the holes through which the tamping bar passed. Courtesy of the Warren Anatomical Museum, Harvard Medical School, Boston.*

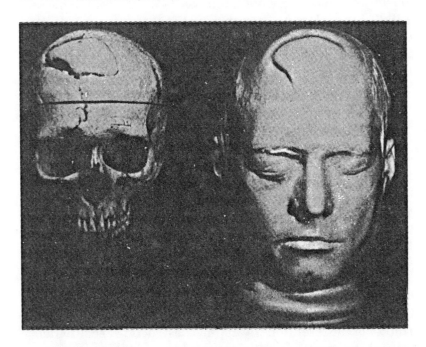

medical accident. A twenty-seven-year-old American, known as HM or Henry M, underwent a brain operation for severe epilepsy. In an attempt to overcome the epileptic attacks, the surgeon removed what he thought was the focal point of the seizures, the hippocampus, of which there is one on either side (see chapter 1). Together, the two form much of the limbic system and lie deep within the temporal lobes (Fig. 4.3 and 4.4).

Previously the hippocampus had been removed from one side of the brains of patients without catastrophic side effects. In HM's case, however, the hippocampus of both sides was removed, with the result that since the operation he has lived, quite literally, from minute to minute. Up until 1953 and the time of his operation, HM's life is still a reality for him because he can remember it; since the operation he retains practically no memories for longer than a few minutes. The reason for this tragic state of affairs is that the hippocampus is essential for the acquisition of long-term memories. That type of operation was of course abandoned, but it made HM into a living guinea pig for neuropsychologists interested in memory.

Neuropsychologist Brenda Milner of the Montreal Neurological Institute has analyzed HM since his tragic operation. From her analyses it is clear that HM is intelligent (his IQ increased from 103 to 115 after the operation), he does well on tests of short-term memory, but his world is restricted to an unlimited array of sequences, each just a few minutes in duration. As soon as one sequence has passed, it is replaced by a new one in which everything has to be relearned. And so the appalling cycle of the temporary is continually re-enacted in the experience of HM.

Loss of long-term memory acquisition inevitably leads to total disintegration of personality, even though limited retention is possible with some simple tasks. HM is unable to remember a person from one day to the next. Even Brenda Milner, who has spent so much time with him over the years, is a complete stranger to him. Each meeting is as if it were the very first occasion on which he has encountered her. HM is unaware of the day of the week or the year, or even his own age. He is unable to say where he works or lives, or how he travels to work. Each time he reads a magazine, it is always as if it were his first glimpse of it. He can assemble the same jigsaw puzzle over and over again, with no hint that he recognizes it.

Since only his memory is affected, HM is aware of his hideous time-encapsulated isolation. He is quoted as saying on one occasion: "Right now, I'm wondering. Have I done or said anything amiss? That's what worries me. It's like waking from a dream; I just don't remember." More philosophically, he is said to have commented: "Every day is alone in itself, whatever enjoyment I've had, and whatever sorrow I've had."

Surprisingly, perhaps, HM is able to learn new skills of movement and works successfully in a rehabilitation center (Fig. 3.4). His deficiency lies in remembering the new content of his conscious experience. That in itself is significant because normal human existence includes building up patterns of experience and appropriate responses to them. Those patterns, laid down in our brains, provide us with a way of conducting life. J. Z. Young calls those patterns "Programs of the brain," because they provide information stores not only for such mundane actions as eating and sleeping, but also for more complicated features of living such as loving and hating, knowing and thinking and even believing and worshiping. Without a long-term memory, therefore, one can have no plans for action, so that an individual like HM is in no way equipped for the ongoing task of coping

*Figure 3.4   Illustration of a test used on HM, demonstrating his ability to learn new skilled movements. Adapted from Colin Blakemore,* Mechanics of the Mind *(London: B.B.C., 1977), p. 95. Based on results of research by Dr. Brenda Milner.*

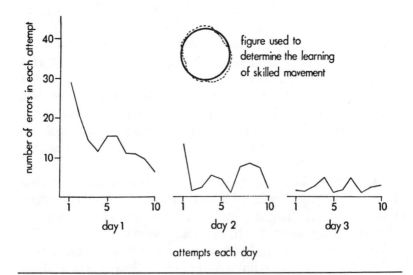

with the demands of living.

*Case 3.* Sublieutenant Zasetsky is one of the most poignant examples in all neuropsychological literature of the tragedy and pathos of a brain-damaged individual. Zasetsky's tribulations and courage have been brilliantly recorded in his own diary accounts and brought to public attention by Alexander Luria in the book *The Man with a Shattered World.*

On 2 March 1943, twenty-three-year-old Zasetsky was participating in the Russian offensive against the Germans in the Battle of Smolensk, when he was hit in the head by a bullet. From that day onward he became a different person. In many respects he had been killed, because his existence thereafter became a kind of half-sleep. In his own words: "Again and again I tell people I've become a totally different person since my injury, that I was killed on 2nd March, 1943, but because of some vital power of my organism, I miraculously remained alive. . . . I always feel as if I'm living out a hideous, fiendish nightmare—that I'm not a man but a shadow, some creature that's fit for nothing."

The head injury which led to that feeling of despair and helplessness affected the left temporo-parieto-occipital region of the brain (Fig. 3.5). It was followed by a prolonged coma and was further complicated by inflammation that produced brain and meningeal adhesions. The result was irreversible damage to the temporo-parieto-occipital region of the left cerebral hemisphere and the formation of scar tissue which produced a partial atrophy of the medulla (Fig. 1.9 and 1.10).

In Zasetsky's case the clinical consequences of the lesions were manifold, affecting his vision, body image, perception of space and reading ability. However, because his frontal lobes escaped damage, he was (and still is) trenchantly aware of his fate. Initially he was unable to perceive anything, his world had collapsed into fragments. His brain was incapable of constructing complete pictures while, to complicate matters even further, the right side of everything was

*Figure 3.5   Side view of the left cerebral hemisphere to show the region damaged in Zasetsky's brain.*

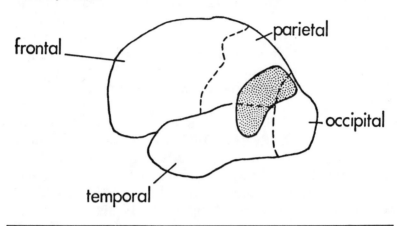

nonexistent. He was left with the unenviable task of attempting to assemble the fragments he saw and guess the objects to which they belonged. Allied with the loss of the right side of his world was the additional loss of the right side of his own body. He simply could not see it.

To make matters worse, his sense of his own body had also changed. Not only was he unable to *see* the right side of his body, he was *unaware that it even existed.* Sometimes he would have the terrifying feeling that his head had become inordinately large or his torso extremely small, and he would even forget where parts of his body were or what was the function of some of his organs. Accompanying the bodily aberrations were spatial aberrations; he had forgotten how to shake hands or what to do with a needle and thread. He found that he had forgotten the names of common objects, and would repeatedly get lost even in rooms and towns with which he had previously been familiar. The difficulty lay in his having lost any sense of space, so that he was unable to judge relationships between objects. Alexander Luria understated Zasetsky's predicament when he wrote: "Confronted with obstacles at every turn, the simplest, most commonplace matters became painfully difficult." Perhaps more horrendous than the other tragedies for Zasetsky was the realization that he was now illiterate. Before his head injury he had been a fourth-year student at a polytechnic institute, but afterward he could read nothing. In his diary he put it like this: "When I look at a letter, it seems unfamiliar and foreign to me. But if I strain my memory and recite the alphabet out loud, I definitely can remember what the letter is."

Zasetsky is not unique. Many others have suffered the sort of injury he endured—in the form of an external injury, from the growth of a tumor, or from some cerebrovascular accident. What is remarkable about Zasetsky is his immense determination to transform his restricted existence into a meaningful life. To do so he set out to learn to read and write in spite of his major visual and orientation limitations. Letter by letter, word by word, he very gradually progressed, forgetting as he went along, reading and rereading and finally writing in an automatic fashion. To give point to such immense effort, he devoted his time to writing a journal of his "terrible brain injury." For twenty-five years he toiled day after day, sometimes devoting an entire day to completing just half a page. Sometimes he would ponder over a page for a week or two. After twenty-five years he had put together a 3,000-page document which he could not even read without enormous toil and perseverance.

Living in a world of undeciphered images, without a past and with no understanding of anything scientific or abstract, Zasetsky's determination to live—as he put it—without a brain, was possible only through the writing of his journal. In it he revived the past in an attempt to insure a future. It was his reason for living because, as he wrote his story, he hoped to overcome his illness and perhaps "become a man like other men." Writing became his only way of thinking. "If I shut these notebooks, give it up," he wrote, "I'll be back in the desert, in that 'know-nothing' world of emptiness and amnesia."

Zasetsky has both succeeded and failed. His reason for

living has enabled him to live, but his deficiencies are as great as ever. There is no ultimate way out for him. His story has no end because the mental stagnation can never be dispelled. Yet one or two of his faculties have remained largely unimpaired: his vivid imagination and his sense of melody. Together they have afforded him some respite from a world otherwise lacking in meaning and coherence.

## Organization of the Cerebral Hemispheres

In order to make sense of these and certain other brain lesions, we need to investigate further the way in which the cerebral hemispheres are organized. Some of their essential features have already been outlined in chapter 1 (Fig. 1.12 and 1.13).

The visual, auditory and olfactory areas are examples of sensory areas in the cerebral hemispheres. Generally, when those areas are depicted in diagrams or referred to in descriptions of the brain, interest centers on the *primary* areas. Around each primary area there is a *secondary* area, however, and outside that, a *tertiary* area (Fig. 3.6). An appreciation of the secondary and tertiary areas surrounding each primary sensory area helps to sort out the weird combination of symptoms demonstrated by Gage and Zasetsky. HM's symptoms following the removal of all his hippocampal tissue are easier to elucidate, since the cerebral hemispheres are not involved.

In the cerebral hemispheres, each primary area receives a sensory input and sends its output only to its own secondary area. There the output is spread out, with each neuron of the primary area being connected with many other neurons widely scattered throughout the secondary area. The difference between the primary and secondary areas can be illustrated by considering the consequence of applying an electric shock to the areas. When done in the primary visual area, a person sees glowing points, circles and fiery tips; by contrast, a shock in the secondary visual area produces complex patterns and even complete objects such as trees or a

Figure 3.6   *Relationship between the primary, secondary and tertiary areas of the sensory regions of the cerebral hemispheres, together with their principal roles.*

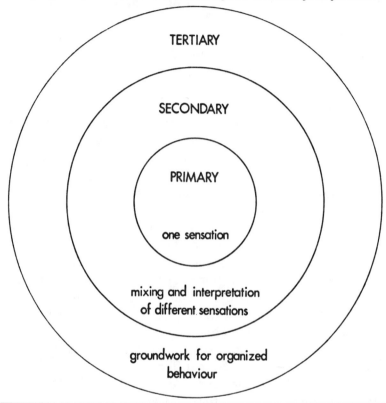

TERTIARY

SECONDARY

PRIMARY

one sensation

mixing and interpretation
of different sensations

groundwork for organized
behaviour

friend. The converse is that, when the primary visual area is destroyed, blindness ensues; when destruction is localized to the secondary visual area, the patient can still see but is unable to put together the individual features of objects to form a whole. Such a person suffers from *visual agnosia*, being unable to deduce the meaning of the image on the retina.

The organization of the secondary areas opens the way for the mixing of sensations, a process which is carried much further by the fact that each primary area is not devoted exclusively to its own sensory input. For example, visual stimuli affect not only the primary visual area but also the primary auditory areas; an auditory stimulus may affect the primary tactile area in addition to the primary auditory area; and on and on. It is not possible, therefore, to isolate one area from another conceptually; when isolation occurs through some brain lesion or other, the effect will likely be a complex and weird intermingling of a number of sensations.

One other point about these areas: each secondary area appears to be mainly concerned with *interpreting* the sensation received by the primary area. In other words, the primary area sorts and records sensory information, whereas the secondary area organizes the information further and codes it. For instance, if the auditory association area is damaged, in addition to the effect on hearing, deficiencies in speech, writing and reading occur. The exact nature of the deficiency will depend on the site and extent of the lesion, but the general deficiency is one of *aphasia*. The patient may hear words but not understand them, or perhaps may be able to write but not read. Such disabilities reflect the connections between different association areas and also between them and the motor areas.

Beside the primary and secondary areas, there are also *tertiary* ones, where data from different sources overlap and lay the groundwork for organized behavior. Those areas bring together visual, motor, and auditory-vestibular inputs. Consequently, damage to tertiary areas prevents the brain from combining those inputs into a coherent whole, with the result that one's world becomes fragmented. The tertiary areas are of particular importance in the production of language, which is fundamental to perception, memory, thinking and behavior. Damage to the tertiary areas of the left cerebral hemisphere, therefore, is especially serious, since linguistic skills and hence the ability to think are disrupted. Such persons may find their inner world fragmented, as they search endlessly for words and ideas, but cannot adequately express themselves or communicate in any meaningful fashion.

*Figure 3.7  For patients with visual agnosia, outline drawings are difficult or impossible to decipher when covered with lines.*

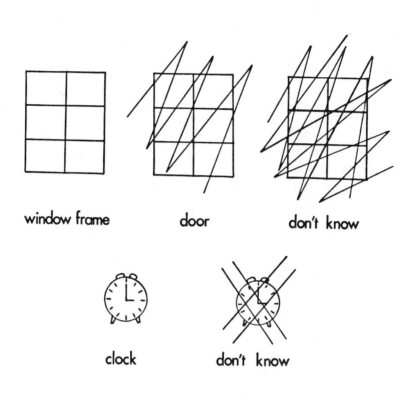

window frame       door       don't know

clock       don't know

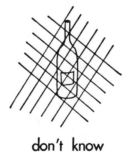

don't know

## Examples of Brain Lesions

*Example 1.* A lesion of the *secondary visual area in the occipital cortex* (Fig. 1.13 and 3.5), as we have seen, produces visual agnosia. Vision is limited to individual features of the total world, but the ability to put them together to form a whole is impaired. Patients with visual agnosia may be unable to recognize a pair of spectacles because of their inability to make sense of the two circles, the two rods and the crossbar. For such patients those may add up to a bicycle. Then again, a telephone with a dial may be mistaken for a clock; difficulties are experienced with outline drawings, and figures covered with lines are impossible to elucidate (Fig. 3.7). Patients with visual agnosia cannot draw properly since they cannot depict an object as a whole—only as a list of component parts (Fig. 3.8). Such patients can see only one object at a time and hence cannot trace the outline of an object or join the strokes together. They either see the pencil and lose the line, or vice versa (Fig. 3.9). From these kinds of evidence, it has been suggested that patients with visual agnosia lack programs for deciphering the code of their own brains.

On the other hand, such patients can recognize objects by touch and can perform a variety of complex intellectual tasks. Interestingly, though, they have difficulty with

*Figure 3.8   Patients with visual agnosia are unable to copy a drawing adequately, since they cannot put the parts together to form a whole.*

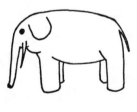
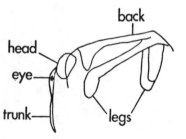

*Figure 3.9   An inability to trace the outline of an object is another feature of persons with visual agnosia.*

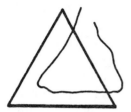 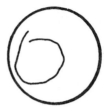

speech codes, such as distinctions between relationships, for example, "brother's father" and "father's brother." Even a localized lesion in the secondary visual area, therefore, has consequences for certain nonvisual phenomena, from which we can conclude that vision (and all it represents in judging distances and relationships) is of widespread significance. At a more general level, we begin to appreciate something of the unity of the brain's programs, a principle we meet repeatedly when dealing with brain lesions.

*Example 2.*  As a second illustration of a brain lesion, consider a local lesion of the *secondary auditory area in the left temporal lobe* (Fig. 3.5). As this is the auditory region (Fig. 1.13), the first noticeable consequence is loss of ability to distinguish clearly between the sounds of speech, a condition referred to as *acoustic agnosia* (sensory aphasia). A lesion on the left side located deep in the temporal lobe may be accompanied by disturbance of audio-verbal memory. Such patients are unable to retain even a few sounds, syllables or words. If asked to remember four words (for example, house —car—bed—field) they may be able to remember only the first and second or the first and last of those words. On the other hand, if the same objects are presented as drawings or even as written words, the patient will have no difficulty remembering them.

Lesions of the secondary zone of the left temporal lobe are, therefore, partial and modality-specific, so that functions localized in other brain areas remain unaffected. In addition to the two disordered features already mentioned, however, other disturbances also occur, including disorders of the understanding of speech, the naming of objects and the recall of words, plus various writing deficiencies. Since the patients are unable to distinguish the necessary acoustic content of a word, they confuse similar-sounding words. The end result is an inability to write words correctly, although they are perfectly competent at copying words—and can even write familiar words.

Put those difficulties together, and the end product is a person with considerable problems of reasoning. Such a brain-damaged person is characterized by a disorderly and highly fragmented way of thinking. Because the various facets making up mental processes are so interrelated, destruction of even one facet has far-reaching consequences for the unity of an individual's personality.

A lesion of the *posterior* zone of the left temporal lobe leads to difficulties in naming objects and also in evoking visual images in response to a given word. Together those difficulties manifest themselves in great difficulty in finding the meaning of a given word. Further, there is gross inability to draw a picture of a named object, in spite of the fact that no difficulty is experienced in copying a picture of it.

Lesions of the *right* temporal lobe have no effect on speech, but apparently have considerable repercussions for musical hearing. For instance, difficulty may be experienced in reproducing rhythmic structures.

*Example 3.* Lesions in the *parietal lobe* (Fig. 3.5) leave vision, hearing and tactile functions intact. What they do, though, is cause disorders of the reception and analysis of information. Patients are unable to grasp information as a whole and have great difficulty fitting together individual components of a single whole structure. Further, they are unable to locate their bearings in space and in particular fail to distinguish between right and left. Inevitably such patients become lost; they are unable to put the appropriate arm into the correct sleeve of a coat; they cannot tell the time if the hours on the face of a clock are not numbered; they cannot find their bearings on a map because they confuse north, south, east and west. In the wake of such deficiencies they suffer from constructional apraxia; that is, they have enormous difficulties in copying letters of the alphabet (Fig. 3.10). Their attempts either bear little resemblance to the original or, if the lesion is less severe, they may draw mirror images.

Depending on the precise location of the lesion in the left parietal lobe, patients may suffer difficulty in grasping logical grammatical structures, being unable to appreciate the meaning of sentences and ideas as a whole. Linked with that is a disturbance of mathematical operations, a symptom referred to as *acalculia*.

Patients with lesions in the left parietal lobe, therefore, experience much frustration in formulating their thoughts and in carrying out complex intellectual operations. Yet their intellectual powers remain largely intact, their ability to describe goals and demonstrate motives still being present. The block comes when they seek to put their plans into operation. We are reminded of the plight of Zasetsky, who demonstrates so clearly the pathological gulf that lies between the integrity of intellectual *activity* and the dis-

*Figure 3.10 Patients with brain damage in the parietal lobe are often unable to copy the letters of the alphabet.*

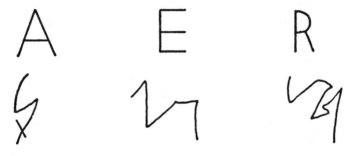

turbance of intellectual *operations*.

This description of parietal lesions has been concerned mainly with the left hemisphere. When we turn to the right hemisphere we find, once again, a completely different set of symptoms. Even large lesions of the right parieto-occipital region leave the higher mental processes intact, so that patients retain the ability to carry out complex logical-grammatical and mathematical operations. They lack awareness of the left half of the visual field, however, and perhaps of the existence of the left side of the body. In writing and drawing, the left side of the page or the left half of drawings will be omitted (Fig. 3.11). Even more remarkable is the fact that the patients are unaware of their mistakes. An additional feature in some patients is loss of a sense of the familiarity of objects, which sometimes appears as a difficulty in the recognition of faces.

*Example 4.* The final example of a brain lesion is that of the *frontal lobes* (Fig. 3.5). Much of our understanding of the important frontal region of the brain comes from removal of the frontal lobes in experimental animals. It was originally pointed out some years ago that, when an animal's frontal lobes are removed, it responds to all stimuli, no matter how irrelevant. Its goal-directed behavior is thus profoundly upset, because it cannot stop itself from responding to irrelevant information. Furthermore, the lack of frontal lobes prevents an animal from correcting any errors it has made.

In humans, the frontal lobes are far more extensively developed than in all other species and are also intimately associated with speech. Since they are implicated in the production of the most complex forms of conscious activity, a lesion of the frontal lobes disturbs the higher forms of voluntary attention. A massive frontal lobe lesion may thus result in a completely passive patient who neither asks for nor seeks anything. A less drastic lesion is more helpful in understanding the consequences of frontal lobe disturbance, because it reveals a disintegration of complex programs of activity and their replacement by more basic forms of be-

*Figure 3.11  Patients with brain damage to the parieto-occipital region of the right cerebral hemisphere often lose the left half of the field of vision as shown in b. which is an attempt to copy a.*

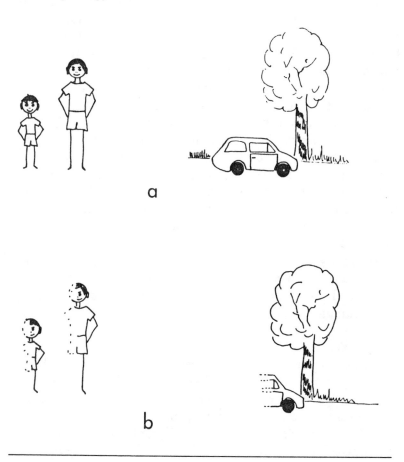

havior. The simpler forms sometimes consist of repetition of stereotyped behavior patterns, neither relevant to the situation nor logical.

These responses, characteristic of "the frontal lobe syndrome," occur when the lesion is in the *lateral* part of the frontal cortex. By contrast, a lesion of the *basal* (orbital) zone of the frontal cortex interferes with olfaction and vision; it also produces behavioral disinhibition and a range of affective disorders including lack of self-control, violent emotional outbursts and related changes in personality. Phineas Gage was an example of that syndrome. A lesion of the *medial* zone of the frontal lobes results in diminished wakefulness, diminished critical faculty and gross disturbance of memory. The overall effect is a state of confusion, with the patient having a profoundly disturbed consciousness, uttering uncontrollable confabulations and showing lack of orientation with respect to the surroundings.

Whatever form the frontal lobe syndrome takes, it includes instability of consciousness and a major unheaval in personality. The relationship of these patients to their world is upset and their grasp of reality is weakened. Destruction of the frontal lobes touches human beings at their most vulnerable point because it places in jeopardy their most precious characteristics. It takes away their ability to select what is important in their environment and then to act on that selection. Lesions of the frontal lobes, even more than the other lesions, bring us face to face with the relation of brain damage to personhood.

## Responses to Brain Damage

Brain lesions of the types discussed above (namely, those affecting various regions of the cerebral hemispheres, especially the cerebral cortex) raise enormous issues. Brain damage may alter a person in profound and far-reaching ways. Apart from any specific impediments present, the person's outlook on life and even ethical standards may appear to be modified by certain lesions. Can people be so radically transformed that they become unrecognizable as themselves?

In most brain-lesioned individuals the changes are for the worse. Their behavioral changes may include a lessening of responsibility and consideration for others and an inability to plan ahead and think in abstract terms. Their lack of foresight and inability to appreciate the rewards or punishments consequent on a given line of conduct will likely lead to unacceptable social behavior. Some authorities, however, consider that even detrimental changes should not be viewed in isolation from the person's previous behavioral traits.

Even undoubtedly pathological behavioral changes are frequently exaggerations of personality characteristics present before brain damage was incurred. Yet it is clear that brain lesions change a person's character for the worse and not for the better. The change is considered by some to be a form of demoralization, an extension perhaps of the sort of demoralization we experience when feeling ill or tired. A major difference is that our illness or exhaustion is generally temporary, whereas a lesion may well have permanently demoralizing consequences.

Expressed in different terms, at least some of the brain lesions considered here bring about the death of an individual's personality—gradually or suddenly, partially or completely. Exactly where the dividing line is drawn along the continuum of personality deterioration and ultimate death is arbitrary and only of theoretical interest. The point is that some cases of brain damage illustrate the death of the personality (in any meaningful sense) without the death of the body. The body is still readily recognizable; the personality on the other hand is a feeble shadow of the personality once known. Indeed, the impoverished personality may be so unlike the original one as to lack essential human and spiritual continuity with it. In that sense, the original *person* may be dead, despite a physiologically intact *body* (with the exception, of course, of the damaged part of the brain).

It is not inappropriate to suggest that brain lesions may to some degree "depersonalize" a human being. A brain-damaged person may cease to be a person in some areas of conduct, the areas dependent on the damaged brain regions. Such an argument has repercussions for our concept of human responsibility. Perhaps a depersonalized individual should not be held responsible for actions governed by the damaged brain regions.

Before rushing to that conclusion, however, we should consider the consequences of treating an individual as less than a person. Zasetsky, with his extensive lesions, would probably have fallen into that category, yet his response to his dilemma bears all the hallmarks of human personhood. Despite grave limitations, his determination to make life meaningful for himself and others epitomizes the human longing to achieve significance. It is unwise, therefore, to discard an individual as a person, even in the face of major brain damage. True, the personality of a brain-damaged individual may be only a dim reflection of what it once was, and the choices open to such an individual may be tragically limited. Nevertheless, as long as some power to choose remains, that individual has not ceased to be a responsible personal agent. The framework of choice may have shifted to something quite unlike the framework employed when dealing with a brain-intact person, but in most instances it still exists. Brain-damaged individuals may have lost much of their freedom, because their injuries may prevent them from attaining the results they intend. As long as some freedom remains, however, the power to choose also remains. If so, brain-damaged persons retain their status as persons, even though the range of alternatives open to them may be greatly narrowed.

The individual and his or her personhood occupy a central position in Christian thinking. In chapters 4 and 5 the significance of the individual person will be seen to be at stake in the face of potentially manipulatory forces. Where brain-intact individuals are exposed to brain-damaging agents, the principle of individual integrity is a relatively straightforward one. In this chapter the extent of responsibility is itself called into question because of the physiological limitations implicit in a damaged brain. Nevertheless, since personhood remains a crucial issue, a Christian would wish to develop what personhood remains rather than dismiss it as of little value. The task becomes one of maintaining and perhaps enlarging whatever individual consciousness remains, as well as defending it from external onslaughts. The issue of personhood will be considered further in chapter 8.

Even if one takes a conservative position, however, some types of brain damage may appear to be so debilitating as to be equivalent to the death of the personality. It may be that we should regard some forms of brain damage as a first installment of death. After all, we tend to do that—without phrasing it so explicitly—with physical impediments, such as severe kidney damage or rapidly spreading cancer. The analogy is limited because of the significance of the brain's integrity for personality expression. Nevertheless, the parallel does emphasize that, in thinking about a person with brain damage, we take as the norm for that person the preinjury personality. The relationships set up while the individual was capable of them, the achievements, accomplishments and perspectives of the individual at that time, must be regarded as the major contributions of that person, representing all he or she once stood for and, no doubt, would continue to stand for were he still in a position to do so.

We have, then, two somewhat diverse approaches to brain-damaged individuals. As far as possible they are still to be regarded as persons, within whatever limitations are imposed by the nature and severity of the damage. Alongside that we need to place an alternative perspective, namely, that the limitations imposed by brain damage constitute a harbinger of death. Brain-damaged individuals need every encouragement to express themselves as fully as possible and, where possible, to utilize undamaged brain regions and hopefully to recover some lost functions. Nevertheless, alongside living with hope must be placed the realization that much has been lost; in that sense, especially with severe brain lesions, a personality that once lived is now dead.

Both Phineas Gage and Zasetsky illustrate the dilemma, Zasetsky perhaps supremely. Both "died" in their early twenties, yet both lived on in a much depleted guise. Which one was the *real* Gage or the *real* Zasetsky? In a way neither was the real one, because both were *aspects* of the former whole person. Both the pre- and post-injury individuals represent Gage and Zasetsky, although the pre-injury representatives show far more clearly the potential of those individuals. We are horrified by what they were after their injuries because we know something of what they were before; after their injuries we compare them to what brain-intact people are like. Our comparisons, therefore, are relative, although we assume that brain-intact individuals tell us something important about how human beings are capable of behaving.

Our expectations of how people should behave raise questions of considerable profundity. We need to ask what we mean by "persons," "consciousness," "normality," "reality." How do we know what the world is really like? Are brain-intact people fully responsible for all their actions under all circumstances? What do we mean by "human responsibility," and to what extent is it dependent on the integrity of the brain? The relationship between the material brain and the immaterial mind continues to challenge us (see chapter 8).

In dealing with a brain-damaged individual, compassion in the face of suffering assumes a major role. An understanding of the theoretical basis for the personality defect is by itself quite inadequate. A *person* with a diseased personality is the object of our interest, not simply a damaged brain. The challenge to Christians in particular, and a challenge we must throw out to society in general, is to show practical compassion for other human beings. Individuals with damaged brains are people in jeopardy, not nuisances to be quietly disposed of or politely forgotten. They are people like us, except that their brains have been partially destroyed. They have suffered one of the consequences of a world in conflict, whether the conflict be political, social or biological. We, too, may one day be victims of that conflict. And we, like they, will be no less human than we are today, in spite of perhaps debilitating limitations. In chapter 6 we shall look at more subtle forms of brain damage from impoverished diets and environments and consider more specifically some principles underlying compassion for fellow humans.

Throughout this discussion our focus has been on brain-damaged adults; no mention has been made of brain-damaged *children*. The principal difference is the possibility for some recovery of function in children; the younger the child, the greater the degree of possible recovery. Generalizations are dangerous because so much depends on the brain region damaged and the extent of the damage. Nevertheless, during the first few years of life when the brain is still growing, "uncommitted" parts of the brain have the capacity to take over at least some of the functions of destroyed regions. For instance, damage to speech centers in the left hemisphere may be partly compensated for by the right hemisphere's acquiring a role in speech. Therapy is thus of considerable importance, particularly in children. Furthermore, it should serve as a warning against discarding even adult brain-damaged individuals as meaningless members of the human family.

A difficulty in dealing with brain-damaged children is our lack of knowledge of how their personalities *would have* developed, had their brains remained intact. The pre-injury personality can be used as a norm only with adults. Apart from its social implications, this problem has repercussions in the spiritual domain. Decisions made by an adult prior to brain injury remain, so that the person who becomes a Christian and later is afflicted by a damaged brain need not fear that his or her relationship to God in Christ is at stake. As Donald MacKay has written, "The events in our lives that have sealed our relationship with Christ are in no way annulled by death. Thus if, through brain damage, the death of our personality takes place by stages, there is no more reason to fear the eternal consequences than if those stages were telescoped into one." He continues: "What matters is always and only the covenant of grace entered into while the personality was entire and undamaged."

In a situation where a person suffers brain injury in early childhood and has to live with the consequences into adulthood, we have to commit that person into the hands of a loving, just and caring heavenly Father—as we do any young child. We can rest assured that whatever responsible decisions can be reached and acted on by such a person are taken into account by God. If no such decisions are possible, God will nonetheless look after such people in mercy and with compassion.

Foundational to every consideration in this realm, whether with children or adults, is the worth of individuals. A brain-intact individual is a single entity which he or she describes as "myself." "I" do things; I decide; I map out courses of action; I have to contend with life and make my own contribution to it. What I am depends on many factors—heredity, environment, a functioning brain. I am a responsible being, with demands made on me and challenges open to me. It is up to "me" to respond and to gain as much relevant information as possible to help me make a responsible choice. If my brain is damaged, I may be less responsible, I may have many fewer courses of response open to me; I may be tragically limited; I may not even be aware of my limitations. Nevertheless, I am still a person; I am a being with whom others must contend. That is why brain damage has so many repercussions, not only for those afflicted, but also for society as a whole.

# 4

## Brain Control

IMPLICIT WITHIN AN UNDERSTANDING of brain functioning and organization is the possibility that the brains of individuals may be controlled by other individuals. That is the context within which "psychosurgery" is viewed by some people.

### The Domain of Psychosurgery

It should come as no surprise that within a technological society biological solutions, which are essentially technological ones, are frequently resorted to in attempts to solve social problems. The distinction between technological and social approaches may actually become blurred in a society molded by technological procedures and thought-forms.

Yet the "new wave" of psychosurgery has created much controversy. To many people it seems to represent a far too efficient tool with which a minority may control and hence manipulate the majority. Consequently, what seems to be at stake is individual freedom—the freedom to be what one is, regardless of the dictates of society.

The use of technologically dependent skills to alleviate suffering and cure specific diseases is one thing, but to assault the brain in an attempt to pacify a violent individual is loaded with social overtones. The logical extension of such a procedure is to intervene earlier and earlier in order to *forestall* possible violence.

The controversy surrounding psychosurgery takes us well beyond purely medical considerations and into medico-legal, ethical, philosophical and theological areas. It highlights the fact that technological answers to traditional questions may be very different from traditional responses. It brings us face to face, therefore, with "technocracy" and its impingement on traditional (often religious) values.

A principal drawback to rational discussion of the issue is polarization of opinion, arising partly out of the emotional nature of the topic. Although individual freedom is a legitimate aspect of the debate, it is not the starting point. Neither is it possible to limit the discussion to medical techniques. The severe consequences of some brain operations and the preponderance of young children and institutionalized patients in some series of cases prevent this.

Christians should not shy away from the issues posed by psychosurgery, but our response also cannot be one of outright hostility. The issues are complex and demanding. They should force us to think hard about our beliefs concerning man—as a person, as a responsible being, as a biological entity, as an interdependent community of individuals, as the purveyor of sophisticated technology, and as a sinner in relationship to the Creator-God. The issues should also drive us to examine the sort of information neurobiologists expect to derive from study of the brain. Even brain research is conducted against a particular cultural background with many implicit expectations, prejudices and limitations.

As a prelude to discussing contemporary psychosurgery, we need to go back to 1891 when a Swiss psychiatrist, Gottlieb Burckhardt, destroyed parts of the cerebral cortex in six psychotic patients. He reasoned that the excitement and impulsiveness of those patients resulted from an excess of neural activity originating in the cortex. Unspectacular results, however, and vigorous opposition from medical colleagues put an end to that initial foray into psychosurgery.

The next episode is better known and was much more influential. In 1935 at an international congress two American neuroscientists described their neurosurgical procedures on monkeys and chimpanzees. By destroying the prefrontal regions, Carlyle F. Jacobsen and John F. Fulton had produced remarkably placid animals. That feature, rather than the learning and memory deficits, impressed a Portuguese neurologist, Egas Moniz, who was in the audience. To Moniz the chimpanzees' behavior before surgery resembled that of many chronically hospitalized mental patients, who were frequently querulous and agitated and in considerable emotional distress. He immediately jumped to the conclusion that brain lesions might be able to calm such patients the way they had calmed the experimental animals.

Within a few months Moniz and a surgical colleague, Almeida Lima, had carried out eleven operations on humans, sectioning the fibers connecting the frontal lobes to the rest of the brain. For that purpose they used a special knife called a leucotome, the procedure itself being known as *frontal leucotomy* or *lobotomy* (Fig. 4.1).

The early results were heralded as a great success and some patients were even described as being cured. In general, agitated, disturbed and aggressive patients became calm and easier to nurse. Some were even able to take part in the social activities of the hospital. The apparent improvement in the mental state of previously psychotic patients led Moniz to hail the advent of leucotomy as a great step forward in the study of psychic functions on an organic basis.

But as time passed and some of the leucotomized patients returned home, it gradually became evident that all was not well. The personalities of many of the patients had been altered in subtle ways. They were less affectionate than they

*Figure 4.1* *Illustration of a leucotome which was used in the classical psycho-surgical procedure of frontal leucotomy or lobotomy. Large tracts of fibers were severed between the frontal lobes and the remainder of the brain.*

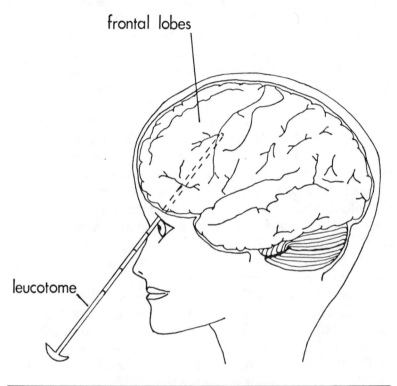

frontal lobes

leucotome

had been and were readily irritated. They found it difficult to concentrate or sustain mental activity. Even more distressing was a disappearance of any social sense or ability to plan ahead. In many instances there was a lack of interest in anything and everything, all meaning and purpose having disappeared from life. Those behavior changes are now referred to as the *frontal lobe syndrome,* characteristic not only of postleucotomy patients but also of brain-wounded patients in whom gross damage has been sustained by the frontal lobes. The predominant feature of the syndrome is loss of many of the finer nuances of personality (chapter 3).

It is regrettable that, in the thinking and practice of many neurosurgeons, the apparent benefits of frontal leucotomy far outweighed its detrimental effects. As a result the operation was performed not only on psychotic patients but also on psychoneurotics and some patients suffering from psychosomatic conditions. The calmness of the postoperative patients, not their apathy, emotional instability, irresponsibility or lack of inhibition, was viewed as of paramount importance. In some instances, of course, the operation proved of considerable help. Nevertheless, its effects were often catastrophic for the integrity of the personality. In spite of such grave drawbacks, at least 50,000 frontal leucotomies were performed in the United States for a variety of psychiatric conditions in the 1940s and 1950s. One American neurosurgeon was personally responsible for more than 3,500 leucotomies. By the late 1950s, mounting concern over the operation's side effects plus the increasing popularity of drug treatments and electroshock therapy, brought that form of classical psychosurgery virtually to an end.

Contemporary psychosurgery has similarities to, as well as differences from, classical psychosurgery. The major similarities are ones of attitude. Surgical approaches are still considered legitimate means of tackling behavioral problems. Moreover, such approaches are regarded as sufficiently specific to solve particular problems of behavior without leaving undesirable consequences for the total personality of the patients. The differences are ones of degree. Instead of cutting many fiber tracts with a leucotome, much smaller, more discrete areas are destroyed by passing electric currents through implanted electrodes. The electrodes, initially used for detecting brain regions with abnormal patterns of electrical activity, are then used to stimulate the tissue with a weak electric current in an attempt to replicate the patient's behavioral response. In that way the abnormal focus in the brain (on the assumption that one exists) can be fairly accurately localized. Associated with the emergence of such

*Figure 4.2 Stereotaxic apparatus used to locate precise regions within the brain. This apparatus can subsequently be employed to destroy those regions via the implanted electrodes.*

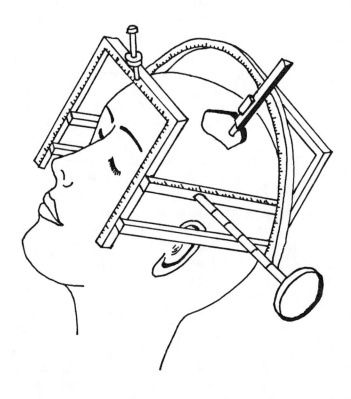

stimulation techniques has been the use of stereotaxic procedures for the accurate and reproducible localization of regions deep within the brain (Fig. 4.2).

Stereotaxic brain surgery has been responsible for a shift of interest away from the frontal lobes, which were the target of classical psychosurgery, to the limbic system. That system is sometimes referred to as the "emotional brain" because, among its many functions, it is implicated in normal emotional responses required for self-preservation. Among the parts of the brain contributing to the limbic sys-

*Figure 4.3 Schematic representation of the parts of the brain constituting the limbic system.*

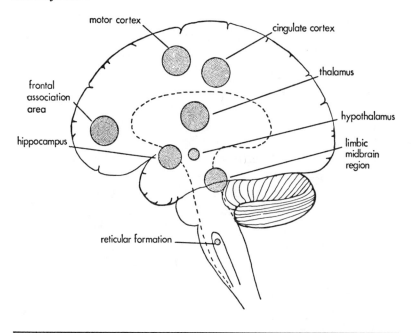

tem are various cortical structures, including the hippo-campus, cingulate gyrus and frontal association cortex, and also deeper-lying structures such as the amygdala, thalamus and hypothalamus (Fig. 4.3).

Surgical removal of parts of the human brain falls into a number of categories. At one extreme are those cases with clearly identifiable physical causes such as brain tumors or head injuries. Surgery to remove or alleviate symptoms arising from such causes has no connection with psychosurgery. In the next category is surgery related to disorders of motor (muscular) function, such as Parkinson's disease. There is reason for believing that destruction of apparently normal brain tissue will alleviate symptoms of the disease. Surgery removes some brain tissue which normally participates in the functions that are disturbed. Although that category borders on psychosurgery, it is not a subject of intense debate. The third category is psychosurgery itself, in which brain tissue is removed in the absence of *any* identifiable physical cause. There is usually some overlap between the latter two categories; in many cases where psychosurgery is contemplated the existence or absence of a physical cause is a highly controversial point.

The various indications for psychosurgical intervention can be divided into two major groups. One group consists of operations to alleviate depression, anxiety and obsessive-compulsive states; the other group is concerned with controlling anger, aggression and sexual problems. It would be unwise to separate the groups widely since some people object to separating them at all; yet it is fair to say that the latter group is the more controversial. It contains the *socially deviant* conditions—anger, aggression and sexual problems—that may reflect the mores of society as much as pathology of the brain.

Although definitions of psychosurgery vary, most construe it as a medical procedure, the principal goal of which is to modify behavior. To some it includes all forms of brain surgery having direct psychological effects. To others it refers to any procedure that destroys brain tissue for the primary purpose of modifying behavior. Others limit it to operations on the frontal lobes or limbic system, the aim of which is to relieve mental conditions in patients with no known brain disease. In practice, psychosurgery must on occasion encompass neurosurgical operations that affect the behavior of patients who suffer from brain disease manifesting itself in epileptic attacks and perhaps extremely aggressive behavior.

### Examples of Psychosurgery
In the United States approximately four hundred psychiatric patients a year receive psychosurgery, a figure that has held since the late 1960s. Of those operations one of the best attested is *cingulotomy,* an operation in which a bundle

of nerve fibers connecting the frontal lobes with the limbic system is interrupted by precise lesions (Figs. 1.12 and 4.1). The principal indications for proceeding with this form of psychosurgery are persistent pain and depression, depression by itself, obsessive-compulsive states, anxiety neurosis and borderline schizophrenia.

In 1976 an American body, the National Commission for the Protection of Human Subjects of Biomedical and Behavioral Research, investigated a number of psychosurgical procedures including cingulotomy. Of eleven patients treated for pain and depression, nine were apparently cured of long-standing illness that had proved refractory to drugs, psychotherapy and electroshock. Five out of seven patients treated for depression alone were markedly improved following psychosurgery. Patients in the other categories were little affected by the operation. It appears that depression, either by itself or accompanied by pain, is most amenable to this form of psychosurgery. The Commission's investigations into other psychosurgical procedures tended to reinforce the conclusion that depression is the one condition fairly consistently improved by psychosurgery. Still, little is known about the rationale behind its effectiveness. It is possible that neurochemical changes occur which alter behavior, or that certain cognitive functions are lost, or that the surgery serves a placebo function.

The other major psychosurgical procedure is not so easy to describe. In fact, it is not a single procedure but a group of procedures characterized by the *reason* for the operation rather than by its *nature*. The reason is a desire to control extreme violence and aggression; the object of the surgery is the limbic system. The area of the limbic system which has received the most attention in regard to violence is the amygdala, a tiny, almond-shaped structure deep within the front part of the temporal lobe (Fig. 4.4).

The basis for believing that the limbic system is implicated in some way in aggressive behavior stems from animal experiments in which that system was either removed or

*Figure 4.4* Positions of the hippocampus and amygdala within the temporal lobe of the brain.

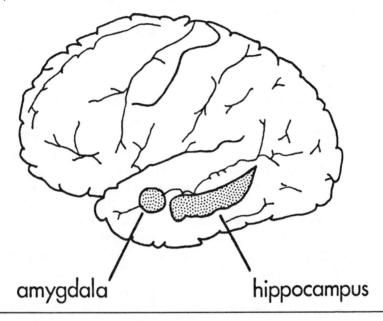

amygdala                                   hippocampus

electrically stimulated. When the limbic system is removed, normally aggressive monkeys or cats have been observed to become placid, are easily handled, and do not respond aggressively even to an attack by other members of their social group. Conversely, stimulation of the system converts a quiet animal into one prepared for attack behavior—as long as the stimulation is maintained. Many studies over the years point toward the same conclusion, that the limbic system in general and the amygdala in particular are intimately associated with the maintenance of violent behavior. That conclusion applies to human behavior as well.

Presenting such a conclusion may suggest that the evidence relating violence to abnormalities of certain brain structures is cut and dried. The situation, however, is not quite so simple. Even a very small area like the amygdala has a number of probable functions, because it makes many connections with other brain regions. That complexity of structure, coupled with the relatively primitive state of our knowledge about the brain, makes for confusion unless great care is exercised in assessing the available evidence.

The decision to use psychosurgery on a human patient in an attempt to control extreme violence is rarely a straightforward one. In many cases the violence is associated with temporal lobe epilepsy (meaning that the seizure starts in the temporal lobe). Further, some of the patients are also severely mentally retarded. Hence assessment of the results of surgical intervention is beset by enormous difficulties.

The drawbacks of using psychosurgery on patients of this type are many. Any connection between violence and epilepsy is murky; indeed, such a connection is rare. There is no concrete evidence that any particular individual's violent behavior is associated with specific damage located in the brain. The fact that amygdalectomy is irreversible and may produce intellectual impairment constitutes a danger of immense significance when contemplating the operation on a mentally normal patient.

Some doctors have suggested that psychosurgery should be extended to patients who are only violent, that is, who have no other medical abnormalities such as epilepsy or even an abnormal electroencephalogram (EEG). At that point psychosurgery takes on overtones of social control, although in the face of mounting opposition to such procedures few psychosurgeons are willing to admit that no brain damage at all is present. More important than polemics is the question of the efficacy of the procedures. Again, the evidence is far from clear. Amygdala lesions (destruction of the amygdala or of portions of it) in some patients have been reported to eliminate or at least diminish attacks of rage; yet it remains far from certain that individuals with a history of explosive violence have specific brain sites triggering violence. Even if they do, are those sites being destroyed by amygdala lesions?

We are still left with the principal technical issue connected with psychosurgery and violence: to what extent does psychosurgery eliminate violence? A neat or even objective summary is impossible. Nevertheless, the conclusions reached by Elliot S. Valenstein in his book *Brain Control* are worth noting. After considering at some length the relation between brain pathology and human violence, he concludes: "Although it is possible that there are more cases of abnormal brain foci triggering violence than may have been suspected, there is little to support the view that this factor is a major contributor to the tremendous proliferation of violent crimes that we are now experiencing."

Because Valenstein's detailed analysis of the results of psychosurgical procedures is characterized by extreme caution and by a reticence to generalize, his conclusions are particularly worthy of note. He writes: "There seems to be strong suggestive evidence (if not absolutely convincing) that some patients may have been significantly helped by psychosurgery. There is certainly no ground for either the position that all psychosurgery necessarily reduces people to a 'vegetable status' or that it has a high probability of producing miraculous cures. The truth, even if somewhat wishy-washy, lies in between these extreme positions."

A task group reporting to the National Institute of Neurological Diseases and Stroke in 1974 ("Brain Research and Violent Behavior") experienced equal difficulty in reaching a succinct conclusion. In part, the report states: "Though most of these (psycho) surgical procedures are reported as successful, the evaluation of the outcome is made difficult because of the following reasons: the diversity of symptoms in patient selection, . . . a lack of detail concerning the degree, character, and thoroughness of the follow up. . . ."

Obviously, much is unknown about the effects of and response to psychosurgery. It may have dramatic results for good; it may not. Amazing "cures" have been reported, but the "non-cures"—more numerous and less amazing—occupy an insignificant place in the report sheets. Psychosurgery is not alone in such bias, but the inability or unwillingness of some psychosurgeons to assess the overall effects of the operations objectively seems endemic. For instance, Valenstein in the early 1970s found that, of 110 American psychosurgeons, only 27 per cent had published their results. Further, of 700 articles reviewed by Valenstein, only 153 contained firsthand data about patients, few of whom had been evaluated by more than three objective tests of intelligence, memory, ability to concentrate or other indicators of psychological capacity following surgery.

The whole realm of psychosurgery is rife with difficulties, uncertainties and contradictions. Not surprisingly it has become a battleground for purveyors of opposing philosophies. The central debate concerns the legitimacy of using psychotechnological tools to modify social attitudes and behavior patterns. The social situation precipitating that debate is the need to control violence.

## The Violence Paradigm

One of the greatest problems confronting the human race at present is the frequency with which violence is resorted to by both individuals and societies. Although this is no new problem for humanity, some of the solutions proposed to combat and eradicate the violent behavior patterns of individuals are new, and they in turn pose further problems. In particular, direct surgical approaches to the brains of violent individuals, even if sometimes successful in eradicating violence, raise such issues as the inviolability of the human person, the reality of human responsibility and the legitimacy of exerting social control through biological manipulation.

In favor of the present "new wave" psychosurgery are Vernon Mark and Frank Ervin, who set the scene for the debate with their book *Violence and the Brain*. Mark, Ervin and their colleague, William H. Sweet, one of a number of groups throughout the world actively conducting psychosurgery, have succeeded in gaining the public's attention with their pronouncements on the potential value of psychosurgery in combatting growing urban violence.

In 1967 the three wrote a now-famous letter to the *Journal of the American Medical Association*. In it they suggested that, in addition to environmental and social factors that were undoubtedly important in the urban riots then raging throughout the United States, a third factor was being ignored. That factor was the possible role of *brain disease,* about which little was known. Consequently, they pointed to an urgent need for research to "pinpoint, diagnose and treat those people with low violence thresholds before they contribute to further tragedies."

The same theme was taken up in greater detail by Mark and Ervin in *Violence and the Brain,* which they wrote in order "to stimulate a new and biologically oriented approach to the problem of human violence." Since they do not present a detailed discussion of social (or theological) causes of violence, it is easy to gain an unbalanced view of their thesis. Essentially, however, they view the problem of human violence as potentially solvable, as a result (one imagines) of biological procedures. Because all behavior filters through the brain (another way of saying "as people think so they act"), they argue that "studying the relationship between the brain and violence is the best way to get to understand the mechanisms of violent behavior."

It is difficult to know how far Mark and Ervin would take that principle, since they readily concede that all violence is not caused by people with damaged brains. They repeatedly emphasize, however, the inadequacy of approaches relying either on the enforcement of "law and order" or on the correction of social injustices; instead, they stress that "many of the individuals who act violently have brain diseases that can be described, diagnosed, treated and controlled."

A significant corollary of the disease approach is a need to detect and treat individuals with malfunctioning brains *before* they commit serious crimes of violence. When psychosurgery is thus advocated as a specific antidote for violence, it becomes a strange amalgam of criminology and "preventive medicine." Viewed in that light, psychosurgery assumes the mantle of the biological answer to social ills, whether imagined or real. If care is not exercised, it could become the ultimate answer to all forms of social deviance; hence the bitter opposition of some to *any* form of psychosurgery.

Although it would be quite incorrect to suggest that all advocates of psychosurgery are prepared to take it to such lengths, serious proposals regarding its use are sometimes startling. Kenneth B. Clark, a social psychologist, put his position in these words:

> Given the urgency of the immediate survival problem, the psychological and social sciences must enable us to control the animalistic, barbaric and primitive propensities in man. . . . We can no longer afford to rely solely on the traditional prescientific attempts to control human cruelty and destructiveness. . . . [Instead we] accept and use the earliest perfected form of psychotechnological, biochemical intervention which would . . . reduce or block the possibility of using power destructively. (Presidential Address, American Psychological Association, 1971)

Opponents of psychosurgery take sentiments of that nature as their cue, and in fear of the *mis*application of the technique reject it in its entirety. The fear most often expressed is that of *social control,* psychosurgery being used for the "good of society" rather than the good of the patient. It is argued by some that doctors have no right to perform operations on the brains of patients in order to make them conform to society's requirements.

That point of view has been forcefully expressed in a number of quarters. A petition produced by an Ad Hoc Committee on Psychosurgery of the National Institute of Mental Health contained this warning: "Since psychosurgery can severely impair a person's intellectual and emotional capacities, the prospects for repression and social control are disturbing."

Peter Breggin, a Washington psychiatrist and one of the foremost opponents of psychosurgery, is more explicit in his condemnation. He opposes all forms of psychosurgery on the grounds that no justification exists for any of the operations and that the procedure has a blunting effect on emotions and thought processes. In short, psychosurgery according to him is an "abortion of the brain" and is being used to repress and "vegetabilize" the helpless, the poor, the institutionalized, women, ethnic minorities and prisoners. In a similar vein, others contend that psychosurgery could be used against dissidents and rebellious groups on the pretext of curbing their antisocial behavior. More specifically, some lay emphasis on the potential threat to blacks in the United States, suggesting that any increased use of psychosurgery will be used predominantly to suppress black people.

The opponents of psychosurgery by and large reject it on alleged ethical grounds, because of its general threat to individuals. The issue of violence as such does not feature highly in their arguments. Proponents and opponents of psychosurgery are thus arguing along rather different lines. Psychosurgery is seen by opponents as a threat to the rights of patients, by placing in jeopardy what they are and may continue to be as human beings. The ethical nature of this opposition stands in sharp contrast to the pragmatic arguments of many proponents of psychosurgery.

As we have already seen, psychosurgery is not a clearcut procedure in any given individual. Violence is not eradicated by destroying the amygdala in the same way that pain is eradicated by removing a diseased tooth. The violence may not disappear; if it does, it may recur. What is more, other aspects of brain function are inevitably affected. The brain is so organized that it is simply impossible to separate any of its functions according to their social implications. The brain is not nearly so simple as some of our cherished ideas. Hence, to suggest that psychosurgery, in anything remotely resembling its present form, is an effective means of social control makes little sense. A dictator wishing to foist his views on society could perhaps do so by using the vast amount of drugs at his disposal. In the world of science

fiction he might resort to psychosurgery, which makes exciting reading. In practice, however, drugs would probably
serve his purpose more effectively (chapter 5).

Yet the argument that aggression, in addition to uncontrollable rage, can be eliminated simply by removing some
brain tissue, has extremely serious implications. That argument is an extreme form of *reductionism,* in which brain
region A corresponds to goodness, brain region B to aggression, brain region C to violence, brain region D to timidity,
and so on (Fig. 4.5). Such a view fails to recognize that each
person is a whole being, made up of and influenced by a vast
range of factors. Among them are the social forces at work
in society. Biological factors (such as brain tumors which

*Figure 4.5  Diagram illustrating the false view that the brain can be subdivided
into discrete areas, A-D, each representing specific qualities. Such a view demands
an organization of the brain that bears no relation to reality.*

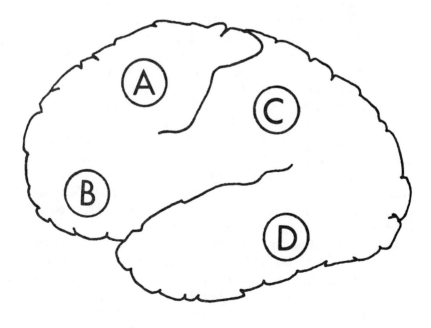

may, under certain circumstances, predispose an individual toward violent behavior) should never be viewed in isolation from social factors (which may predispose a person to violence). One cannot be isolated from the other when deciding which is of paramount importance in a particular individual's violent episodes.

Once some account is taken of the social/environmental matrix of violent behavior, we must consider what Peter Schrag has called "the tyranny of the normative." It is easy for society to erect norms of reasonable conduct and then define as "deviance" any form of behavior significantly different from those. If violence becomes a sign of mental disturbance, the appropriate treatment may be seen as surgical modification of some part of the limbic system. Under that guise, brain technology could rapidly become the solution of choice in dealing with social conflict, whether the conflict is violence, homosexual behavior, hyperactivity in children or drug addiction.

Biological remedies for social problems are no substitute for social solutions. The alleged biological remedies often may not be remedies. Moreover, control of *individual* deviance is no answer to the problem of understanding the various *social systems* of which the deviance is but a part. Careful distinction needs to be made between *deviance* and *disease*. Stephen Chorover, a neurophysiologist, argues that the definition of deviant behavior is essentially social and cultural, suggesting that types of deviance change as society evolves. By contrast, types of biological disease remain constant across societies. Granted that the distinction between deviance and disease may not always be clear-cut, the social context of violence should not be discarded.

Christian counselor Jay Adams argues that all faulty behavior stems ultimately from our estrangement from God. Mental illness has, in a Christian perspective, a theological as well as a medical base. The Christian counselor will, therefore, attempt to discover whether faulty behavior is the result of an organic defect or of sinful actions or both.

Nonorganic behavior problems might stem from sinful life patterns. The emphasis in Adams's approach is that patients be treated as whole persons, who are largely responsible for their behavior even when this is of a bizarre nature.

The significance of this conclusion and that of Chorover is reinforced by analyzing the biological evidence for a relationship between violent behavior and convulsive disorders. A close relationship between the two constitutes the pivotal point of Mark and Ervin's emphasis on the effectiveness of biological solutions. Individuals with poor control of violent impulses are said by Mark and Ervin to be suffering from the *dyscontrol* syndrome, the alleged brain damage affecting the temporal lobes (Fig. 1.12). There is no convincing evidence, however, that cases of episodically occurring violence caused by brain pathology represent anything but an insignificant percentage of societies' violence. And the temporal lobe is not the only brain region in which the damage-violence paradigm allegedly holds. The fundamental difficulty is in demonstrating that brain damage, such as a tumor or epileptic focus, actually *causes* the violent behavior of an individual. Although such damage may sometimes be causal, alternative explanations such as childhood experiences and socio-economic conditions must first be eliminated (Fig. 4.6). Whatever the outcome of the deliberations concerning any particular individual, the person as a person demands adequate consideration.

An interesting question in this context is what we mean when we say that a procedure "works." The answer we give to that question has direct relevance for assessing the outcome of psychosurgery. Has it worked if the patient is rendered more docile and more susceptible to the dictates of authority? Under some circumstances it probably has; under others it undoubtedly has not. Joseph E. Bogen, a neurosurgeon, argues that an individual is better, not when his or her behavioral repertoire has been reduced, but when it has been enhanced. Hence the goal of treatment should, ideally at least, be a more—not less—differentiated person,

*Figure 4.6 Violent episodes may arise from a number of causes, including a brain tumor, childhood experiences and general socio-economic conditions. The cause should not be automatically ascribed to the tumor without taking the other factors into account.*

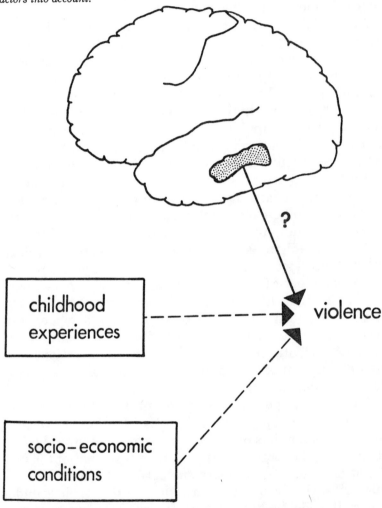

with a greater capacity for choice. This is in accordance with the Christian view that individuals are important in their entirety and in the potential they represent. We should strive for increased behavioral potential and diversity of attitudes, even though the latter may sometimes be a more difficult option than conformity.

In some instances an individual may be so violent and out of control that psychosurgery seems to be the one remaining therapeutic tool. Before a decision is made to proceed with psychosurgery, however, a number of questions should be answered. Will the operation benefit the *patient?* Have *all* alternative forms of therapy been tried? What are the likely side effects of the particular operation? What is the probable cause of the patient's violence—is it definitely brain damage, or is it a psychopathic condition, or might it be spiritual in origin? Is the anticipated procedure in any sense experimental? What is the moral justification for the operation? What moral principle is being appealed to? What other moral principles are relevant?

One further issue is the use of psychosurgery on prison inmates to overcome extreme violence. The question of whether free consent is ever possible under these circumstances is a difficult one. This is because, as Willard Gaylin has put it, "The damaged organ is the organ of consent." Also relevant is the distinction between a prisoner volunteering for an experiment that may help *others* as opposed to accepting a procedure that may directly affect the condition responsible for his own confinement. Even if free consent is not completely out of the question under prison conditions, the forces militating against it are so great as to render psychosurgery on inmates a very unwise procedure.

### Electrical Stimulation of the Brain

Implicit within the psychosurgical procedures considered in the last section is the technique of electrical stimulation of the brain (ESB). When a weak electric current is passed through an electrode placed in the brain, the tissue in the vicinity of the electrode tip is stimulated. Some aspects of ESB were considered in chapter 1 in connection with functional localization in the cerebral hemispheres. Reports of José Delgado and James Olds in the early 1950s on the rewarding and punishing consequences of brain stimulation set modern ESB in motion. To understand its contribution to present-day psychosurgery we need to sketch briefly the results of some of the now-classical experiments.

In 1953 James Olds found that, when certain parts of the hypothalamus in rats were electrically stimulated using implanted electrodes, the rats appeared to enjoy the stimulation (compare Fig. 1.10 for position of hypothalamus in humans). Responding to the shock, the animals soon learned to do whatever was required of them in order to receive it. When the electrode circuit incorporated a switch with a lever the rats could press themselves, they stimulated their own brains regularly and repeatedly. Olds concluded that the parts of the hypothalamus giving such a reaction constituted *pleasure centers*. His findings were interpreted to suggest that the rats derived such pleasure from self-stimulation of their hypothalamus that they continued pressing the lever until they fell asleep or dropped from exhaustion. Regrettably, that simplistic interpretation held almost unrivaled sway for a number of years.

In addition to the pleasure centers, there is evidence that *punishment centers* also occur in the hypothalamus; other centers are apparently implicated in the development of obesity, thirst and hunger. And, of course, there is the amygdala which, when electrically stimulated, gives a variety of reactions including rage (Fig. 4.4).

These conclusions have a veneer of legitimacy. Nevertheless, they leave a number of disturbing questions unanswered. Basically, any results obtained by treating a particular brain region in isolation from other brain systems are bound to present an incomplete picture. They fail to treat the brain and its internal connections as an entity.

Some of the most dramatic examples of ESB are illustrated by the work of the Spanish neurophysiologist, José Delgado. For instance, he reported that a five-second stimulation of a particular spot in a monkey's brain will make the monkey stop whatever it is doing, make a face, turn its head to the right, walk on its hind legs around its cage, climb the cage wall and return to the floor. With cessation of the stimulation it grunts, stands on all fours, and resumes normal activity. Each time the button is pressed the monkey goes through exactly the same ritual. Similarly, cats can apparently be induced into either paroxysms of rage or excessive contentment simply by stimulating the appropriate brain region. In one instance Delgado, with considerable showmanship, went into a bull-ring and stopped a charging bull by stimulating one of its brain regions by remote control.

Is ESB to become the basis of an "electroligarchy," as some have suggested? Is brain stimulation irresistible to the point of self-destruction? Elliot Valenstein has analyzed this and related questions in detail, and he thinks not. The rats so frequently reported as stimulating themselves relentlessly to the point of death are not the automata they are often made out to be. They stop to eat, groom, sleep and even explore the environment. Where rats have starved in that type of experiment, the unavailability of adequate food supplies appears to have played as important a part as the "irresistibility" of the rewarding brain stimulation. Comparable human experiments also present difficulties of interpretation; a number of workers believe that the curiosity of the subjects is a major contributing factor in the results obtained.

Transition from ESB's potential to specific psychosurgery is a key factor in discussions on brain manipulation. Valenstein approaches the matter cautiously, placing due weight on the specificity of ESB. He writes: "It is one matter to appreciate the value of brain stimulation as a basic research tool that provides a means to learn more about how the brain is organized to carry on its many functions, but it is quite another matter to conclude that we may soon be in a position to manipulate the brain and thereby modify human behaviour in a predictable, practical, and desirable manner."

In fact research workers have observed that electrodes that seem to be in the same brain locus in different animals often evoke different behavior, and that electrodes located at very different brain sites may evoke the same behavior in a given animal. It appears to follow, therefore, that in order to understand the precise response of an animal, a knowledge of the brain region being stimulated is insufficient by itself. In addition, some more general factor or combination of factors—perhaps the personality of the animal or its behavioral tendencies—seems to be essential for the formulation of the response. At any rate, it has been found that stimulation of the amygdala may increase aggressiveness and provoke aggressive acts in aggressive patients, whereas similar stimulation in nonaggressive patients may fail to elicit aggressiveness.

It is also important to understand that the behavior resulting from brain stimulation depends on factors such as the expectations of other people, the position of the person in his or her social group and the state of other parts of the person's brain and body. When such environmental factors, plus the frequent lack of anatomical specificity, are taken into account, the significance of a phenomenon may be far less obvious than imagined.

Delgado's famous experiment in which he halted a charging bull in its path by ESB may not be all it is sometimes made out to be. The aggression-reducing interpretation regularly placed on that experiment is open to question. Rather, the fact that brain stimulation affected the movement of certain muscles may overshadow any postulated effect on an aggressive drive.

In summary, brain stimulation is far less predictable than is frequently suggested. The response tendencies of the subjects and their emotional state taken together constitute major determinants of the behavior evoked by stimulation. For Valenstein, there is little justification for the belief that brain stimulation is a valid technique for locating discrete foci that trigger violence. Nevertheless, the ESB technique is in its infancy and in all probability will emerge as a major therapeutic tool (and agent of brain control) in coming years.

Brain stimulation is the basis of present-day psychosurgery, so its further refinement may lead to revolutionary developments in psychosurgery.

## Brain Modification and Personal Identity

Any procedure designed to alter some aspect of an individual's personality immediately raises the question: What *is* a person's real nature? That is not a new question, of course. It has long been known that brain damage or brain disease may alter a person's behavior patterns. With psychosurgery, however, what was previously unavoidable now becomes subject to human control. That takes us to the heart of technological prowess. Instead of living at the behest of his environment, technological man controls his environment. When he strives to control his own brain, psychosurgery comes into its own.

A great deal of thought needs to be given to ways of determining the identity of a person's nature and personality. To what extent do they depend on the brain's physical integrity? An allied question concerns the definition of *normality*. How do we know when an individual is normal, that is, normal within the limits of his or her own personality? And to what extent is normality determined by social, rather than biological, expectations?

Those are vital questions in the context of violence and psychosurgery. It is essential that we distinguish between "normal" and "pathological" anger, since the latter could conceivably render an individual liable to psychosurgery or some other form of medical treatment, whereas the former does not. That raises again the fundamental question of whether a malfunctioning brain or the dictates of society constitutes the hallmark of pathogenicity.

Deeply personal considerations enter at this juncture. What possibilities are opened up by psychosurgery in alleviating disturbing conditions such as severe depression or extreme violence? On the assumption that psychosurgery is capable of, for example, converting violent individuals into quiet, law-abiding ones, such conversions may be construed as of benefit to the community, to the individuals themselves and also to their families. But what is meant by "benefit"? What is gratitude in this instance? Is our chief consideration the individual himself or those around him and society at large? Donald MacKay puts his finger on one of the critical issues when he writes: "The difficulty is that the man to whom we are currently answerable, when considering whether or not to perform the operation, is the violent person we want to change."

The success of psychosurgery, in whatever terms it is being judged, depends on altering the decision-making organ of the person concerned. Except for those who adopt an extreme dualist position (chapter 8), this fact poses immense problems for all operations directed at modifying social behavior patterns. The conflict is essentially between maintaining the personality of the individual regardless of destructive social consequences, and of modifying the personality in an attempt to render the individual more acceptable to society's expectations.

When the conflict is expressed in rigid terms, people are forced to take unwarranted, extreme positions. In a Christian perspective what emerges as of supreme importance is the *good of the individual person,* not the inviolability of personality nor the comfort of society. To undervalue human life in its wholeness and in its spiritual and social interrelations is to underrate the meaning of individual humans in God's sight. Furthermore, it negates the Incarnation by suggesting that human life is unworthy of Christ's high estimation of it. *Human dignity* is a facet of human personhood bestowed on us by God in creation and redemption. Accordingly, individual humans are to be respected, not because of any functional value they may have in society, but because of what they *are* as human beings. Helmut Thielicke describes this as their "alien dignity," based as it is on God's view of them and his sacrifice for them in the life and death of Jesus Christ.

The integrity of "personality" is important but its importance does not override other features of human life, such as the ability of individuals to fulfill themselves, to aspire to wholeness, to experience the inner freedom to be and to love. There may be some instances where psychosurgery can actually enhance features characteristic of human existence. Even if that is true, however, it must be remembered that brain operations *destroy* tissue and so destroy connections between one group of structures and another.

Whatever the validity of the above points, they are based on an assumption that the essential identity of the person is retained. But what of an operation that may destroy brain structures essential to the continuity of personal identity? Is that equivalent to terminating the life of one individual and introducing another, quite alien personality? Perhaps. If so, the Christian concern would then be whether the change in personal identity outweighs the detrimental effects of the behavior disturbances on the person as a responsible and responsive human being. A complete loss of all sense of personal identity must be equated with the death of the person. Could it ever be morally right to induce such death of personhood deliberately to overcome social problems? The closest analogy may be the death penalty for serious crimes, an issue on which Christians are divided. Even this analogy, however, is inadequate since it refers to physical death, unlike psychosurgery with its separation of physical and personality death.

In practice, such extremes are rare as a consequence of psychosurgery. Far more frequently, psychosurgical procedures probably bring about exaggerations of personality traits present before the operation. Awareness of those effects, however, requires constant monitoring; the probability that most psychosurgical procedures will exert at least some influence on the total personality and behavior of the individual calls for serious thought and responsible decision making.

It may be essential to distinguish between psychosurgery

in its tasks of remedying medical defects and alleviating suffering on the one hand, and of attempting to improve an individual's capacity and potential on the other, at least as a guiding principle. For Christians (and many others), realization of an individual's full potential is a goal for which to strive, although all that the term "full potential" encompasses is far from clear. Whether psychosurgery will ever have a part to play in this is equally unclear. For the present our aim should be the development and realization of the capabilities of individuals, which follows from our acceptance of people as creatures in God's image.

An allied question raised by psychosurgery is that of *human responsibility*. Are we always fully responsible for all our actions? Are there ever any exceptions? Sooner or later we are confronted by those individuals with brain damage (or genetic abnormality) which appears to diminish their *degree of responsibility* as normally conceived. In *some* individuals at least, there is a connection between the extent of their responsibility and the state of their brains, so that "full" responsibility becomes an arbitrary term.

Great stress has sometimes been laid on such a connection, as in those persons with the XYY chromosome abnormality. The extra Y chromosome has often been indicted as a cause of antisocial behavior and criminal tendencies. Some years ago after a few accused murderers were reported to have the additional chromosome, the inmates of prisons and mental institutions were vigorously tested for that abnormality. By implication, possession of the XYY chromosome pattern would divest a person of responsibility for certain criminal acts. On carefully comparing XYY males with controls from the same subpopulations, however, no major differences in personality characteristics as measured by various psychological tests are evident. Although the XYY condition is peripheral to the psychosurgery debate, it underlines the necessity of viewing individuals as total people and not as isolated chromosomes or disembodied brains.

If psychosurgery is contemplated to combat violence, it must first be determined to what extent an individual is *responsible* for that violence. If it appears that he or she is responsible for it, psychosurgery would be a gross infringement of God-given rights, even if the individual is abusing those rights. Alternatively, if there are clear indications that the violence is a direct result of some brain pathology, treatment of that pathology is a means of rectifying something which itself is interfering with a God-ordained pattern, namely normality.

In practice the choice is not always clear. Strictly speaking, the treatment of a pathology removes the operation from the realm of psychosurgery. More important, it may not be possible to decide whether the pathology is actually the *cause* of the violent behavior. So, is the individual responsible for the violence or not? When the answer to that question is shrouded in the mist of ignorance, the responsibility of doctor to patient comes to the forefront—and that is no less a God-given responsibility.

It would be easy to dismiss psychosurgery out of hand, as the tip of the iceberg of the *technocratic control* of the human brain. But is that sufficient ground for dismissing it? If so, much else within our society should be similarly dealt with. In the hands of some, psychosurgery is an example of extreme *reductionism*. Yet it may also be viewed as a necessary part of the treatment of the whole person in a few exceptional cases.

What humans can do to other humans by way of psychosurgery rightly alarms us. But parents cripple their children emotionally and spiritually every day by neglect, selfishness and cruelty. Psychosurgery needs to be seen in perspective. There is no doubt that it raises issues of exceptional significance, taking us deep into the realms of human responsibility and freedom. Yet psychosurgery is not alone in doing that, as the next chapter will demonstrate.

# 5

## Behavior
## Control

IN THE LAST CHAPTER we explored the most explicit but least widely used method of behavior control, psychosurgery. For the sake of convenience it was referred to as *brain* control because it is a direct approach to the brains of individuals. Psychosurgery, of course, can also be regarded as a potent form of behavior control.

With the present chapter the emphasis shifts away from direct brain control to other methods of behavior control. We must not forget, however, that the brain will always be the mediator in any behavior modification. Of the two issues to be considered, use of pharmacological agents and psychological conditioning, the former stands at the dividing line of brain/behavior control; the latter emphasizes educational techniques rather than access to the brain. Together with psychosurgery they can be seen as a continuum in the process of brain/behavior control.

## Pharmacological and Psychological Engineering

Before confronting the worlds of drugs and conditioning, let us consider their contemporary social significance. Tranquilizers will serve to introduce the drug realm through the following testimony:

> I take Librium because it takes me out of reality and into a make-believe world where my hands don't tremble, my cheek doesn't twitch, and my stomach is released from an iron band of nerves. With the help of the drug I am able to cope with the pressures and the fast flow of work. If I didn't take Librium I would probably become an alcoholic, and then I couldn't work at all. Without tranquilizers a working day becomes an ordeal I have to brace myself to face, my nights are sleepless and life is unbearable.

Those are the words of a thirty-two-year-old administrative executive, words that portray the feelings of millions of people throughout the world both in the inadequacy they represent and in the solution adopted to overcome the inadequacy. The tranquilizer is perhaps the supreme symbol of our day. People expect to feel strained, but instead of reaching for an aspirin (the cure-all for headaches) they now reach for Valium or Librium (the cure-all for life's troubles). The inroads of an impersonal, technological society are matched by the phenomenal success of the "minor" tranquilizers as panaceas for all sorts of anxiety and depression. The impression is easily gained that good health is impossible without tranquilizers, and normal life is only attainable when discomfort, unhappiness and anxiety have been banished by one tranquilizer or another.

A revolution in attitudes is under way. Its starting point is mass indulgence in tranquilizers, although other types of drugs are also a part of it. Before considering them in detail, we should note that drugs such as tranquilizers exert their effects on our brains and hence on our personalities. As a result they have a potential for modifying our perception of reality and our response to it. That potential has implications for our way of life and far-reaching consequences for society. It forces us to think seriously about what constitutes contentment, normal human existence and fulfillment in life.

Alongside drugs we have the technology of conditioning, which Perry London, professor of psychology and psychiatry at the University of Southern California, sees as perhaps the main problem area of behavior control. Conditioning methods combine some of the precision of drugs or surgery with the pervasiveness of education. Such methods are administered, quite literally, from the first days of life. Since they resemble the means by which all human beings learn their emotional attitudes and skills, the behavioral consequences of conditioning are very difficult to eradicate. With such permanence, coupled with its noncoercive nature, the potential of conditioning, becomes enormous.

Because of that potential, a Roman Catholic ethicist, Father Bernard Häring, contends that a major area of manipulation is provided by the fields of learning and education. The options open to educators are clearly delineated by Häring: one possibility is to conceive and carry out education after the pattern of animal management; the other is to direct it purposefully toward insight, motivation, goodness, a holistic view of life and the development of concern for the freedom of all people. Hence a developing child will be treated either as an object to be managed or as a partner in a process of growth. The first mode of practice is a one-way relationship in which reciprocal openness is shunned; the second is a true dialog situation, the level of dialog depending on the maturity of the child.

These issues will be considered in the latter part of this chapter. First we will look at drug-related methods of behavior control.

## The Psychotropic Maze
Psychotropic drugs exert their main effects on the nervous system and are employed for that reason in psychiatric treatment. Tranquilizers are but one example of these mood-

affecting drugs. Although one is startled by recent developments in psychotropic drug use, it is well to remember that
drugs of that nature have been used by the human race for
thousands of years. They form an integral part of the culture
of most societies. For instance, hashish was used by the
Assyrians as long ago as the eighth century B.C. The preparation of opium is described on clay tablets by the Sume-
rians at about the same time. Coca leaves, the source of cocaine, have been chewed by millions of Peruvian Indians
since before the Middle Ages. These examples reflect the
antiquity of drug usage as well as the long-standing dependence of humans on drugs that affect their brains.

As we come nearer to our own day, we find examples of
people concerned with the effects of mood-affecting drugs on
both themselves and others. The best known is perhaps
Thomas De Quincey who, in 1821, wrote a book with the re-
vealing title, *Confessions of an English Opium Eater*. Toward the latter part of his life, English novelist Aldous
Huxley made repeated journeys into drug-induced mysticism and set in motion one of the earliest of the contemporary drug-centered vogues. Huxley's *Doors of Perception*,
published in 1954, may be a modern classic but it finds its
place in a well-worn, ancient tradition.

The truly scientific side of the history of mood-affecting
drugs commenced in the 1890s and came to public attention
in the 1940s and '50s with the synthesis of LSD and the first
of the modern tranquilizers. As far back as Victorian times,
however, drugs such as chloral and paraldehyde were employed to sedate psychiatric patients. In the early 1900s the
*barbiturates* started coming into clinical use as antidotes to
anxiety. Before long it was realized that they are highly addictive. The brain becomes habituated to them, so that ever
larger doses are required to produce the same effect. Prolonged use of barbiturates leads to chronic intoxication,
severe deterioration of the personality and inability to function adequately in society. In the United States, according to
Hordern, 10,000 deaths from barbiturate poisoning occur

each year. In the United Kingdom, half a million people use barbiturates regularly; 110,000 are chronically dependent on them, and over 1,500 people use them each year to commit suicide.

Barbiturates are hypnotics, agents that depress the nervous system. Although they are gradually being replaced as sedatives, they remain of major social importance. Unfortunately, their value in reducing anxiety is bought at a high personal and social cost.

The barbiturates have proven to be the forerunners of the major social phenomenon of the psycho-pharmacological scene, the tranquilizers. For practical purposes, tranquilizers are subdivided into two groups: the minor ones which are widely used in the general community, and the major ones which tend to be used only in serious psychiatric conditions.

The first of the *minor tranquilizers, meprobamate (Miltown),* appeared on the market in 1955. Unlike sedatives, tranquilizers exert a calming effect, allaying anxieties and tension without depressing the level of consciousness or alertness. Although meprobamate is still marketed for the relief of anxiety, it has been largely superseded by a group of drugs known as the benzodiazepines, of which by far the best known members are *Valium (diazepam)* and *Librium (chlordiazepoxide).* With these two drugs, which came on the market in the early 1960s, we are confronted by the tranquilizers in all their alluring efficacy.

Valium and Librium provide pharmacological tranquility on demand, with relative safety, effectiveness and few side effects. True addiction is very rare, and overdoses are seldom fatal. Their disadvantage is that they may be used as a substitute for facing life's problems. It is easy for a busy physician to prescribe a tranquilizer rather than attempt to solve the underlying conflicts causing the anxiety and depression. Often the solution to a person's problems lies in discussion and sympathetic counseling; when these are not possible or convenient, tranquilizers serve as a technological solution. As a short-term method of alleviating acute distress and as a prelude to counseling, these drugs have an important role in modern therapy. But when employed as long-term solutions to social situations, they introduce other problems, not only in the medical area but also in philosophical and theological realms. Psychological dependence on them (as opposed to physiological addiction) is frequent; as dependence increases, the doses escalate and the prospects of a social solution diminish. Bad side-effects of minor tranquilizers include confusion and temporary memory-loss, especially among people over sixty years of age.

To sketch the almost universal acceptance of the minor tranquilizers is to enter the realm of astronomical figures. Somewhere around twenty million Americans take either Valium or Librium, with well over eighty million prescriptions being dispensed annually (Fig. 5.1). Over half a billion dollars is spent each year on Valium alone in the United States. In the United Kingdom, over one million people take Valium or Librium either regularly or intermittently. What is true of these two technologically advanced nations is also true of others. Furthermore, consumption of these drugs is increasing steadily, an indication of the pressures of technological societies and of doctors' prescriptive responses to them. In Australia, for instance, there has been a four-fold increase in the number of prescriptions for these compounds per 100 persons over the years 1971-75.

At the level of society in general, there can be no denying the enormity of the impact of the minor tranquilizers. Almost every individual has either taken a tranquilizer for a period or had a close family member take one. That is not true for the *major tranquilizers,* although their impact on psychiatric practice has been no less dramatic. Chlorpromazine was first introduced in the early 1950s and within ten years had been given to an estimated fifty million patients to control psychotic disturbances. The major tranquilizers, generically called phenothiazines, are widely used for con-

*Figure 5.1  Trends in the usage of psychotropic drugs between 1965 and 1970 in the United States. From M. B. Balter and Jerome Levine, "Character and Extent of Psychotherapeutic Drug Use in the United States," a paper presented at the Fifth World Congress of Psychiatry, Mexico City, 1971.*

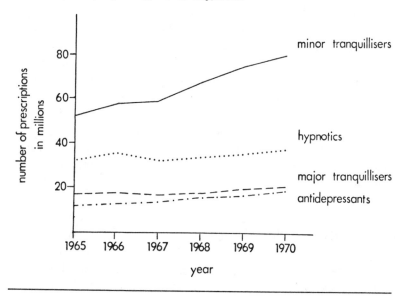

trol of schizophrenia and for neurotic patients with marked agitation. Phenothiazines have powerful actions and bring about a pronounced reduction in levels of anxiety, excitement and aggression. Introduction of this group of tranquilizers has been largely responsible for reducing the number of long-term patients in psychiatric hospitals, replacing them by short-term patients who are often able to be released and to hold down jobs in society and lead a semblance of a normal life.

Tranquilizers calm a patient but do not elevate his or her mood. *Stimulants,* such as the amphetamines ("purple hearts"), do. Initially used as an antidote to depression, the amphetamines were widely administered in the 1950s and '60s. Marketed in a variety of forms (Benzedrine, Dexedrine,

Methedrine), they appear to increase alertness, confidence and decisiveness, counteracting fatigue and drowsiness. Given intravenously, they lead to pleasurable "highs." They are highly addictive, and chronic use may lead to psychosis and permanent brain damage. At the height of an amphetamine craze in the 1950s, there were half a million addicts in Japan. One feature of amphetamine-taking is reduction of appetite, so amphetamines have been and still are prescribed for would-be dieters. Weight-reduction requires long-term use, with attendant danger of addiction, since the appetite returns to its previous level once the drug is stopped. When mixed with barbiturates, amphetamines become far more dangerous, with vicious withdrawal symptoms and severe effects on the brain.

One cannot consider amphetamines today without reference to their use in treating *minimal brain dysfunction* (hyperactivity). That phrase is applied to children who are clumsy and inattentive at school, and who are frequently impulsive and disobedient. According to some authorities, as many as ten per cent of American children fall into that category. Although behavioral disorders are ascribed to the hyperactive condition, most children diagnosed as suffering from hyperactivity have no known damage to the brain. Brain dysfunction is suggested by the child's behavior, and that alone is regarded as justification for large doses of an amphetamine. In view of the known harmful results of prolonged amphetamine administration, the treatment is a matter of concern to many people. Amphetamines do quiet the child, often in a dramatic manner. But the issue is whether drug administration is the appropriate response to naughtiness in difficult-to-control children, since the drug produces an alteration of the brain. Assessment of the social milieu of the child may reveal that the behavioral problem is a response to a bad environment, malnutrition or an unhappy family background. To ignore such possibilities in favor of an explanation related to brain mechanisms is to underrate the complexity and significance of the individual person. It is not even clear why amphetamines appear to quiet rather than stimulate young children. Doubt that amphetamines are an appropriate remedy for hyperactive children in the long run has led to current efforts to find dietary answers for the problems of such children.

Another group of psychotropic drugs is the *antidepressants.* In some ways we are on surer ground with them. Principally employed in medical practice, they are safer than other psychotropic drugs. They do not produce euphoria or lead to addiction. Although withdrawal symptoms are not experienced, the patient's depression may return when administration of the drug is cut off. The most valuable of the antidepressants are the tricyclic compounds, of which imipramine (Tofranil) and amitriptyline (Elavil) are the best examples. These antidepressants have largely replaced another group, the monoamine oxidase (MAO) inhibitors, which had dietary and other interactions.

Even with the new antidepressants, however, there are side effects, including extreme dryness of the mouth, constipation, disorders of vision, impotence and muscular weakness. Minor as such problems may be, compared with severe depression, they cannot be ignored.

Before leaving these drugs, it should be pointed out that even the best ones do not actually "cure." If the social conditions precipitating the reaction remain, the person's maladapted response will recur. What the drugs achieve is alleviation of symptoms, an important achievement for someone in a desperate state of tension and anxiety. Since they exert their effects principally by altering patients' moods, they have little, if any, influence on the information content of the brain. In other words, they are instrumental in altering, even temporarily, the way in which a person views and responds to the world. Nevertheless, one's actual relationship to that world remains unchanged. Rarely, therefore, do drugs constitute the sole therapeutic approach to psychiatric illness, because they generally leave untouched the cause of mental disturbance.

## Nonmedicinal Tranquilizers

Strictly speaking, the drugs to which we now turn are not tranquilizers in the narrow pharmacological sense. Nevertheless, to the extent that they shelter people from the ravages of life, they undoubtedly serve a tranquilizerlike function. Two such drugs have an enormous impact on Western societies. They are alcohol and nicotine.

Why is it appropriate to call alcohol and nicotine "tranquilizers" and "drugs"? Both help relieve tension and anxiety and play a role in dispelling nervousness. These are characteristics of a tranquilizer. In addition, one of the serious drawbacks of alcohol and nicotine is also associated with tranquilizers—drug dependence. In social terms, therefore, they are tranquilizers. It is almost self-evident that they should be described as drugs, since they have well-recognized pharmacological properties. Regrettably, the common practice is to reserve the term *drug* for socially unacceptable preparations such as LSD, heroin, cannabis and the amphetamines. Such agents are regarded as harmful, in contradistinction to more socially acceptable substances: barbiturates, minor tranquilizers, many analgesics and, inevitably, alcohol and nicotine. To make such a distinction is dangerously inaccurate and misleading. Most of these preparations affect the brain and modify a person's response to surroundings and responsibilities. Although their effects on the body vary, a distinction based on social acceptability is worthless.

Taken together, alcohol and nicotine are probably the most dangerous drugs used in the Western world. That is not to say that they are more dangerous to individuals than, for example, LSD. They are not. But when their rate of consumption is taken into account they become a problem of gigantic proportions.

The major problem with alcohol is *alcoholism*. Of those who drink socially, approximately one in seven becomes dependent on alcohol, producing the major drug-dependence problem of contemporary society. Early symptoms of alco-

Figure 5.2    A graph showing the results of a study in which the risk of having an automobile accident increases as the blood alcohol level increases. Courtesy of Robert K. Borkenstein, Indiana University Center for Studies of Law in Action.

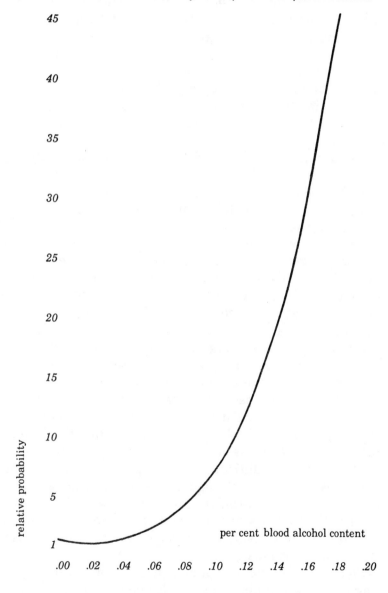

holism are social ones, including socio-marital problems, difficulties at work, traffic accidents (Fig. 5.2), debts and aggressive behavior. Physical complications are seen only after the condition becomes advanced, with liver complaints and nervous system and psychiatric afflictions predominating. Alcoholics are found in all social strata. Many professional people who become alcoholics have had previous histories of outstanding accomplishment.

One estimate of the number of alcoholics worldwide is one per cent of the population. The social problem becomes more real, however, when we consider a highly technological society like the United States. From figures quoted by Hordern it appears that in 1974 of those Americans over the age of eighteen who drink alcohol, approximately ten per cent were either alcoholics or problem drinkers. Even more telling are the social consequences of the drinking, which accounts for over fifty per cent of traffic fatalities and a similar proportion of murders; it increases the likelihood of separation or divorce by seven times and decreases life expectancy by at least ten years. In financial terms its cost in the United States has been put at fifteen billion dollars each year. Unfortunately, the absenteeism, reduced efficiency and accidents contributing to that figure wield less power in government planning than the eighteen billion dollars that alcohol brings in annually in taxes.

Alcohol has long been the most common self-prescribed remedy for anxiety and depression. With the onset of heavy drinking, however, further anxiety is generated and, in its wake, self-reproach, isolation, depression, impaired judgment, violence and difficulty in holding down a job. A vicious circle is established, with ensuing personal degradation that far outweighs the initial tranquilizing role of the alcohol. Admittedly, that description is extreme; nevertheless, it is a common enough result, with personal and social consequences of enormous dimensions.

*Cigarette smoking* has much in common with alcohol usage. Both are promoted as desirable adjuncts to sophisticated living. Ubiquitous advertising of cigarettes and liquor fosters tacit approval of particular lifestyles; the emphasis is always on leisure, romance, adventure and social success. Cigarette smoking allays anxiety and provides some instant relief of tension. For millions of people, the immediate gratification must seem worth the risks associated with smoking.

The dangers of cigarette smoking are well known. Death rates in cigarette smokers are 30-80 per cent higher than in nonsmokers, while morbidity rates are far in excess of those of nonsmokers. Deaths from cigarette smoking are enormous; for instance, in Australia in 1979, between ten thousand and twelve thousand deaths were caused by cigarettes against seventy deaths from illegal drugs. The extent of the smoking habit is immense, with around 600 billion cigarettes being consumed each year in North America. Smoking does not cause the type of personality deterioration seen in alcoholism, yet it shortens life, precipitates lung and heart ailments and leads to a general lowering of physical well-being. That seems a high price to pay for tobacco's alleged tranquilizing properties. Once again, an attempt to cope with anxiety by pharmacological means alone leads, on a long-term basis, into a cul-de-sac.

## Hallucinogens

With hallucinogens we return to the psychotropic drugs. The hallucinogens, variously known as "psychotomimetics" or "psychedelics," fall into the mind-expanding category. They include naturally occurring substances such as cannabis, cocaine and the mushroom derivative, mescaline (Fig. 5.3). Of the synthetic substances, LSD is by far the best known. In general, both groups of hallucinogens produce distortions of mood, perception and thought processes. From a social standpoint, cannabis and LSD together constitute a striking contemporary symbol of defiance of the standards of conventional society. The spiritual consequences of that rebellion will be discussed in chapter 7.

Figure 5.3  Plants from which psychotropic drugs are derived: a. female mari-juana plant; b. ergot-infested rye seed (LSD is synthesized from an alkaloid in ergot); c. peyote cactus, from which mescaline is derived.

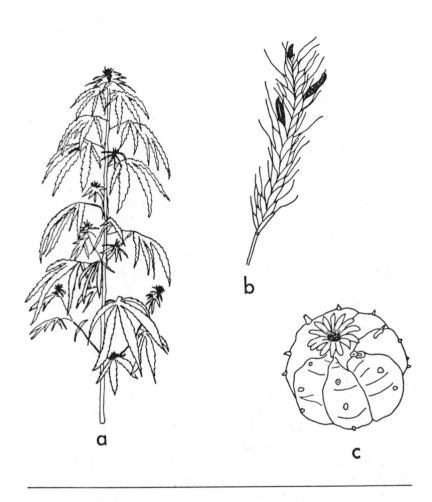

*Marijuana* (cannabis, "pot," "grass") may be smoked by as many as 300 million people throughout the world. Perhaps as many as 10 million use it regularly in the United States. Even in the face of severe penalties, its usage has escalated considerably in technologically developed countries. Among the dominant motives for taking it are curiosity, bravado and desire for its effects, which include euphoria, increased sensory awareness and a feeling of well-being. Smoking marijuana in the United States has definite overtones of defiance toward parental authority, the law and the establishment. With the young it also reflects the pleasure of participating in group activities, where it serves much the same role as alcohol. Many young adults who regularly use marijuana appear to do so to help them cope with the exigencies of normal existence, just as many adults indulge in minor tranquilizers and barbiturates.

The dangers of regular marijuana use are still ardently debated. Adverse effects mentioned in studies include the onset of psychosis, although that is probably rare. Escalation to other drugs and aggressive behavior due to marijuana alone are probably equally rare. More relevant are certain associations of marijuana use. For instance, in one investigation in Melbourne, Krupinski and Stoller noted that only eighteen per cent of heavy users of illicit drugs confined themselves to marijuana. Most users also indulge in other drugs and may be heavy drinkers and smokers. Becoming a marijuana user may indicate commitment to an outlook and lifestyle based on acceptance of drug-induced excitement, relaxation and mental stimulation. Lack of interest in conventional goals and a general lethargy and lack of motivation may be inherent in that outlook.

Acceptance of marijuana as an intimate part of a lifestyle denotes withdrawal to some degree from the world of outer reality to the private world of inner experience. Since that inner experience is in part drug-dependent, the escape from reality cannot be lightly dismissed. It needs to be emphasized, however, that the experiences generated by marijuana depend very much on the expectations of the users. Anticipation of a "high" or of a mystical experience is almost a prerequisite for such experiences from smoking marijuana. Any assessment of the psychological and social consequences of marijuana use, therefore, cannot be based solely on the pharmacology of the drug.

With *LSD* (lysergic acid diethylamide, "acid") we enter the realm of true psychedelic drugs and a major channel through which young people have sought new kinds of mind-revealing experiences. The world of LSD is a world of transcendental experiences, drug-induced mysticism, open-ended adventures of the mind and revolutionary bohemianism. At the height of the LSD phenomenon in the 1960s, Timothy Leary, ex-Harvard professor and psychedelic guru, saw LSD as ushering in a religious renaissance. For him and many of his followers, the LSD experience was a deeply spiritual event, a maelstrom of transcendental visions and hallucinations. The intense sensory experiences were interpreted as providing insights into new realities, opening up vistas normally repressed and leading to deeper understanding of the universe. For Leary, the only way to these expanded frontiers of consciousness was through the psychedelic drugs: by "turning on, tuning in and dropping out."

The LSD philosophy says that, in order to advance, our nervous systems must be modified so that we become more aware of what we are "on the inside." Reality lies inside our heads; it is in our perceptions, which therefore become all-important. The irony of mystical-chemical explorations is that, in attempting to become part of some cosmic unity confined-to the world of sensory impressions, Leary and others like him made themselves utterly dependent on drugs, which are very much outside our heads. Drug-induced experiences are transitory; when they pass, they leave nothing but a memory of hallucination. Satisfactory religious or even mystical systems cannot be built out of sensory fantasies.

Like other psychotropic drugs, LSD affects the mood of an individual. Unlike most of the others, it affects perceptions and sometimes produces hallucinations. In some instances, it gives rise to a pattern of behavior superficially resembling certain psychoses, notably schizophrenia. The reactions of different individuals to LSD ingestion vary widely, depending on personality, expectations and the circumstances under which it is taken. Unstable individuals have, on occasion, committed suicide under its influence or, assuming they were immortal, have indulged in feats ending in death.

Among the behavioral consequences of LSD ingestion are perceptual changes, including distortions of size and perspective, increased brightness of colors, intensification of sounds, and actual changes in the body image. Reactions to these changes vary from one extreme to the other. To some they are heaven; to others, hell. For some there is transcendental bliss; for others, a paranoid world of hideous evil. Thought processes are similarly affected. Some individuals feel that thoughts are rushing headlong into and out of their heads; others sense that their thinking is slowing to a halt. Regardless of those differences, however, efficiency in performing intellectual tasks is severely affected.

In spite of poor memory and diminished powers of concentration, LSD users feel that their work is of a high standard, higher than under normal circumstances. That feeling applies particularly to creative work, although it has more general applicability. Hence LSD use is advocated by certain artists and writers. Even that claim appears deceptive, though; it is highly unlikely that psychedelic drugs can provide a shortcut to creative talent (Fig. 5.4). Perhaps that aspect of the LSD cult is symptomatic of all its facets: it is deceptive in holding out the tantalizing hope of a new cosmos and a new consciousness when, in fact, there is only the old cosmos and the old consciousness. There is no new understanding or new awareness, only sensations and feelings coupled with a dangerous drug cult rebelling against the mores of conventional society.

The psychological effects of "dropping acid" (taking LSD) are sometimes quite devastating, although less predictable than the effects of "shooting" heroin (diacetylmorphine, "smack," "horse"). Heroin and morphine, narcotics derived from the opium poppy, are the characteristic "hard" drugs, capable of producing true physiological addiction. The ef-

*Figure 5.4 Comparison of drawings before and after LSD ingestion. From H. Goodell et al., "Studies in Human Cerebral Function: the Effects of Mescaline and Lysergic Acid on Cerebral Processes Pertinent to Creative Ability,"* Journal of Nervous and Mental Disease, *122 (1955), 487-91. Used by permission of The Williams & Wilkins Co., Baltimore.*

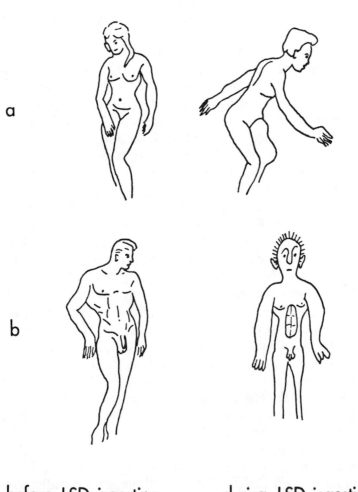

a

b

before LSD ingestion          during LSD ingestion

fects of LSD are often milder and more predictable than those of PCP (phenylcyclohexylpiperidine, "angel dust"), a drug capable of producing severe dependence (if not true addiction) and of turning some people into virtual zombies, others into raging psychotics.

## From Psychological Malaise to Mood Control

The taking of certain drugs is readily accepted by society and is endemic within society. In highly developed technological societies, alcohol, nicotine, the minor tranquilizers and the barbiturates fall into the accepted category; marijuana and the stimulants are also accepted in the eyes of many younger people. LSD is not quite in that category but, along with the other hard drugs, finds acceptance in a substantial subculture. Most of the other psychotropic drugs, which are more or less restricted to medical use, are less likely to become major influences on a society's lifestyle. Of course, patterns of drug abuse change rapidly in a changing society; the United States has seen heroin use expand from the urban ghetto into middle-class suburbia, cocaine become a sophisticated "party" drug, and PCP, once used only as an animal tranquilizer in veterinary practice, manufactured in illicit laboratories for sale on the streets. Law enforcement procedures and legislation to control abuse both struggle to keep up.

In other societies other drugs, even opium for instance, may be endemic. Factors responsible for such variation in drug usage include the availability and degree of acceptance of a drug. Analyzing the pattern of drug usage in a society may provide insights into the pressures, aspirations and beliefs of that society.

Drugs form an integral part of the life of most societies, ranging from the ordinary citizen's bottle of sedatives to the addict's craving for alcohol or heroin. However innocuous or degrading their superficial appearance, the ordinary citizen and the addict are both part of our drug-based psychochemical society.

Before focusing on the issue of excess drugtaking, we should not overlook the contribution of psychotropic drugs to the alleviation of mental illness. Indeed, they have played an important part in gaining an understanding of psychiatric conditions such as neuroses and have also made immense contributions to the treatment of organic conditions such as Parkinson's disease. Drug therapy to rectify brain disease has been a major achievement of psychopharmacology, for which we should be grateful. Concern is not centered on that type of drug usage, but on the wholesale administration of psychotropic drugs for those with no major brain disorders or with no brain disorders at all. Regrettably, distinctions in this realm are sometimes quite arbitrary. Discretion must be exercised in deciding whether social or medical forces are determining the approach adopted.

In spite of legitimate contributions of psychotropic drugs to psychiatry, questions remain. Is widespread usage and ready community acceptance of any psychotropic drug a matter for concern? Could such a trend be essential for the stability of a technologically oriented society? To what extent have psychotropic drugs radically altered lifestyle and even fundamental human attitudes?

The main demand for psychotropic drugs stems from a sense of inadequacy to cope with life's stresses. Modern urban society is characterized by impersonality, boredom, loss of purpose in life, a sense of being lost in a technocratic, machine-dominated age, a sense of frustration at being unable to find fulfillment in traditional roles within family, community or workplace (Fig. 5.5). The list could be prolonged. Each facet reflects some aspect of a society undergoing rapid change.

Whatever the diagnosis of our society's needs, however, the remedy adopted has been the increasing use of mood-affecting drugs. Thus, rather than trying to modify society, it has been accepted as a *given*. Individuals who find themselves unable to cope with the demands of this society alleviate their plight by modifying their own reaction to circum-

*Figure 5.5 Illustration of the age and sex incidence of endogenous depression in an English community. The highest incidence occurs in the forties and fifties, with far more females being afflicted in these age groups. Adapted from C. A. H. Watts,* Depressive Disorders in the Community *(Bristol: John Wright, 1966).*

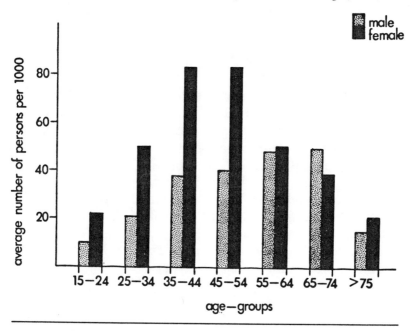

stances. They do that by drug-induced modification of their brains. The inordinate taking of tranquilizers probably has greater consequences for mankind than the more restricted use of hard drugs.

Such an analysis, which sounds alarmingly like George Orwell's *1984,* is in fact the reality of today. The only difference is that, whereas *1984* probably horrifies most people, our present psychochemical society is readily accepted. Even if some modification of brain responses is considered desirable, what we are seeing is a society based on brain modification as *the* solution of choice for individuals under normal circumstances. In that regard, a psychochemical society is fundamentally new and different from any previous society.

Of course, the sort of brain modification brought about

by most of the psychotropic drugs differs from psychosurgery in that it is temporary. Although drugs and psychosurgery must not be considered on a par for that reason, drug dependence and drug addiction must not be overlooked. These are capable of transforming temporary structural effects into functionally long-term effects.

Some people fear a totalitarian foisting of mood-affecting drugs on the population, which is a possibility. But the frightening actuality is widespread *voluntary* taking of psychotropic drugs as a means of escape from the difficulties of the real world. Although some of the drugs are highly useful in certain circumstances, their overindulgence has become a means of shielding people from pressures they need to face up to and, if possible, resolve.

Drugs are modifying behavior patterns more profoundly than we generally realize. We keep looking for technological rather than social solutions to our problems (see chapter 4), and it is usually easier to prescribe drugs to alleviate symptoms than to tackle the social situation giving rise to the symptoms. Some use of drugs is undoubtedly justified within a stringently controlled therapeutic framework, but dependence on drugs by an increasing number of people and by society as a whole leads to a change in the quality of life. Our lifestyle is being revolutionized; people no longer seek the resources to overcome difficulties and despondency as beings created by God. Rather, accepting their situation in a fatalistic spirit, they then modify their reaction by chemical means.

Are we not thus undervaluing the significance of the human person? In the Christian perspective, human beings reflect certain essential characteristics of God: we are rational and responsible, with a knowledge of good and evil; we have freedom to follow what is good or, alternatively, what is evil; we are aware of God in a general religious sense and have immense potential for developing our humanness. Hence we are responsible to face up to life as it is and, in responding, to mature as a human person. Choice and suffering are integral aspects of the human situation, and to flee from them is to be diminished as humans and to reject the reality of an inherent aspect of a fallen world.

The question that arises over minor tranquilizers and similar drugs is the degree to which they shelter people from the reality of God's world which, because of the Fall, is also a world of sin, suffering and fear. Suffering as a total phenomenon cannot be eradicated by biological procedures; psychological trauma is no exception. It can frequently be relieved by various forms of therapy, but undue reliance on psychotropic drugs leaves the human problem untouched. To alter people's neurological responses by such drugs is to admit that their suffering is insurmountable. It tacitly identifies them as machines to be manipulated bit by bit. It ignores them as creatures made in God's image and designed for his glory and happiness.

In Christian terms, each individual must be treated as a unity, as a being with God-directed relationships, with person-to-person obligations, with family and social responsibilities, with physical and spiritual dimensions, with hopes and aspirations and fears. We should not be surprised that, living in a highly impersonal and technocratic society, many find difficulty in coping with the pressures of alienation. Our response should be a deeply sympathetic one. Our efforts should be directed toward restoring those personal and spiritual relationships that lie at the heart of a God-centered universe, rather than manipulating the brains of the afflicted. Our response should enlarge the conception of what it means to be human, not concede that human beings are merely an amalgam of physical components.

Our technological society has given us the ability to perform astounding feats of biomedical manipulation. In principle, they have immense potential for restoring damaged personalities to some semblance of normality. Yet to depend on biomedical intervention as a routine part of normal existence is to limit ourselves to the capabilities of human ingenuity. Implicit in that course of action is acceptance of human autonomy and rejection of the sovereignty or even relevance of God.

As God's creatures we have freedom, though in this fallen world our freedom is restricted. To accept dependence on psychotropic drugs as a norm is to embark willingly on a lifestyle that limits our God-bestowed freedom even more. True freedom entails accepting God's gift of freedom in the person and work of Jesus Christ and working out that freedom through the opportunities and strife of human living. Lifestyle is a religious issue. To what use will the human race put its psychopharmacological abilities?

The "brave new world" is already here, having quietly overtaken us. We face not a few controllers who dispense mood-affecting drugs on an unwilling populace, but a populace that demands the drugs. For the foreseeable future, ordinary citizens will continue to determine how much interference they will tolerate to their brains and behavior patterns. In the final analysis for most people, we ourselves will decide how we want to use our own brains.

## Psychological Conditioning

Although psychological issues are outside the realm of this book, some attention must be paid to "conditioning" as an extension of the forms of brain and behavior control already discussed.

Some writers use the terms "behavior control" and "manipulation" interchangeably, one definition being "the changing of environmental conditions to which an organism is exposed so as to bring about a definite behavioral result." That definition is favored by Christian psychologist Gary R. Collins, who points out that the result may be production of new behavior, maintenance of existing behavior or elimination of undesirable behavior. Collins considers three manipulation devices to be particularly powerful and potentially dangerous: sensory deprivation, psychotherapy and conditioning. Conditioning will be discussed here and sensory deprivation will be mentioned in connection with states of consciousness in chapter 7.

Two major forms of conditioning paramount for any discussion of behavior control owe their genesis to Ivan Petrovich Pavlov and B. F. Skinner, respectively. In the 1920s the conditional response studied by Pavlov was applied to the learning of emotional behavior in children; that application led to a suggestion that many fears and phobias are, in reality, emotional reactions learned by conditioning. If so, the reactions should also be amenable to treatment by conditioning procedures. In the intervening years many problems have been tackled by conditioning techniques, including bed-wetting in children, asthma attacks and alcoholism.

Alongside the conditioned response of Pavlovian "classical conditioning" may be placed the "reinforcement conditioning" derived from the laboratory studies of Skinner. As its name indicates, this method of conditioning relies on the reinforcement of behavior patterns by certain means. For instance, acceptable behavior can be reinforced by administering a pleasing response—food, a smile or some other reward—whereas undesirable behavior can be suppressed by withholding the appropriate form of reinforcement. In that way it is possible to change the behavior of uncooperative children; patterns that have been altered include thumbsucking, stealing, tantrums, stuttering, hyperactivity and social withdrawal. In adults, reinforcement conditioning has been employed in the treatment of overeating, neuroses, phobias and various sexual behavior patterns including homosexuality.

These two forms of conditioning confront us with behavior-control technology in its essence. A vivid, idealized picture of a society run along such lines is provided by Skinner in his famous novel, *Walden Two*. Skinner proposed that children be systematically controlled by conditioning procedures in order to teach them self-control. The underlying principle emerging from *Walden Two* and other writings by Skinner is that satisfactory social organization depends on optimum use of the possibilities of behavior-control technology.

Potential conflict comes to the fore when behavior control is applied in the treatment of mental illness and crime (if one considers that crime can be "treated"). These areas of social deviance require value decisions about the respective importance of individual freedom of action and the dictates of society. The question of social deviance arose in our discussion of psychosurgery; it emerges again, perhaps in a more acute form, in any consideration of conditioning as a means of behavior control.

Perry London pinpoints the ethical dilemma of behavior control when he writes: "The values which promote the maximum use of conditioning technologies, and the values which the maximum use of those technologies in turn promotes, are those of reducing individual pain and of enhancing the sense of self-control, that is, of personal freedom, in people's lives. That sense comes, however, from being satisfied with one's behavior, not from being capable of altering it." Tensions are inevitable when an individual's wishes are at variance with those of society and when society expects individuals to contribute to its general welfare. The ability of society to put its wishes into practice by having its psychologists use behavior-control technology converts any theoretical consideration into harsh practical reality. Today's control methods are so effective that it is no exaggeration to speak of "the engineering of consent." The significance of this discussion goes beyond mental illness and crime, impinging on all traditional concepts of personal responsibility and political freedom (Fig. 5.6).

There is no way of escaping these dilemmas. Individuals live within society; society, in order to exist, must have accepted standards and hence obligations. But what standards, and in what manner and to what degree are they to be imposed on individual members of society? The question, according to Perry London, is how much power over their own behavior must the good society vest in each of its members, and at what risk to its own integrity.

Most viewpoints on behavior-control technologies seem

*Figure 5.6  Relationship between the individual and society, outlining the issues raised by modification of the brain in response to society's demands.*

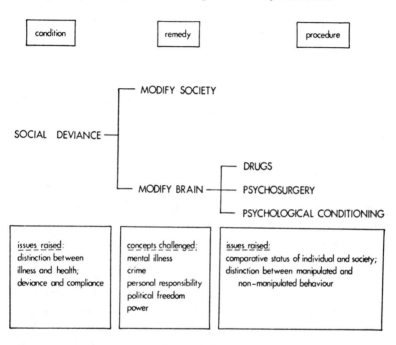

imbalanced, either in the direction of support or opposition. For example, there is the "Leonardo da Vinci syndrome," the cynical name given to the phenomenon of frequent diagnoses of schizophrenia for political dissenters in the Soviet Union. One of the earliest people to be diagnosed in this way was the well-known biochemist and gerontologist, Zhores Medvedev, who in 1970 was confined to a mental hospital for engaging in two unrelated activities, gerontology and social criticism. The use of psychiatry as a political weapon radically alters the nature both of political debate and of behavior control: dissident behavior becomes the product of an unbalanced mind—which is diagnosed solely on the basis of dissident behavior. Aware of the possibilities inherent in such gross abuse of psychiatry and, in particular of conditioning technologies, a vocal school of antipsychiatry has arisen.

Perhaps even more extreme in their emphases, proponents of the antipsychiatry position, spearheaded by psychiatry professor Thomas Szasz, argue that mental illness is a myth and not a medical condition. According to Szasz, disease can affect only the body, so there is no such entity as mental illness. It follows by impeccable logic that, if there is no mental illness, there can be no hospitalization, treatment or cure for it. Mental illness is not, in that scenario, something a person has, but is something a person *does* or *is*. Consequently, psychiatric diagnoses are stigmatizing labels, phrased to resemble diagnoses and applied to persons whose behavior annoys or offends others. In a somewhat similar vein Jay Adams argues that wrong labels of behavioral responses lead in wrong directions. Hence the importance of distinguishing between psychiatric, medical and theological labels and their respective solutions.

Such extreme views help us characterize the incipient fear of behavior-control technologies. The focal point of both reactions centers on the demands and expectations of society (Fig. 5.6). Once society becomes all-important and the individual is relegated to the status of a conforming cog, behavior control gives those in authority the tools to control others. Under such state domination, the behavior modifiers rarely question the legitimacy of that authority or the means by which they exercise it over deviant individuals. On the other hand, to dismiss mental illness as a concept in no way solves the problems raised by misuse of behavior-control techniques. It may even insure that they are employed under unregulated conditions. The antipsychiatry school, by emphasizing the sickness of society and the political side of psychiatry, forfeits any scientific basis for psychiatry and shows only limited concern for the human side of an individual's illness.

Deviance from the mores of society cannot, by itself, amount to mental illness. It has nothing to do with brain pathology and may have nothing to do with inappropriate responses to one's environment. Where it is seen as mental illness, it is probably society's perception of appropriate conduct that is at fault; the environment may be pathological. The dilemma is to decide whether or not society's expectations are pathological; this is a social and ethical decision, not a medical one. While mental illness is undoubtedly a valid concept, the task of demonstrating its legitimacy in the absence of recognizable brain pathology is hazardous.

We are still left with questions about the way society will cope with the vistas opened up by behavior-control techniques. Theologian Allen Verhey has expressed the issues raised in these words: "You cannot have a morally satisfactory social system unless you make morally reasonable use of behaviour control technology." His statement, pinpointing the importance of this form of technology, also stresses the moral commitment that must undergird it. Perry London has also put forward several propositions concerning behavior-control technology as a means of social control. He regards social deviance as more defensible now than at any previous time in history. Since most of the ethical and legal problems revolve around practical definitions of crime and mental illness, London thinks that the range of behaviors potentially subject to behavior-control technology could be reduced simply by redefinition. Finally, he argues that a liberation ethic may sometimes contribute less to individual happiness than an ethic of "benevolent coerciveness."

Perhaps the line between certain types of illness and health is not so clear-cut as frequently imagined (Fig. 5.6). Similarly, the distinction between social deviance and compliance with the wishes of society is, under some circumstances, rather flexible. Further, it may not always be possible to distinguish between manipulated and nonmanipulated behavior. Sociologist David O. Moberg has pointed out that all human beings are controlled to a very high degree. If that is so, how can control be entirely deprecated? Moberg thinks that order in society, though maintained by compliance is a basic prerequisite to freedom even though it limits freedom. It is perhaps ironic that techniques that can enslave people can also free them to live happier, more fulfilled existences. For instance, reinforcement techniques may transform people into robots but, used more appropriately, they enhance educational learning processes. The distinction between enslaving and liberating techniques lies in their goals and in the dialog built into them. Where no dialog is possible, manipulation will likely be the end result. Where human beings are viewed as means to an end rather than ends in themselves, behavior-control techniques are likely to be enslaving. The manner in which they are employed is closely linked with the theological presuppositions of the controllers.

Even when limited by social controls, individuals, as beings formed in the image of God, are in a position to decide between the limited alternatives open to them. That is another way of expressing the fact that human beings are not just passive victims of social pressures. Rather, we are in a position to respond to social pressures and to decide which options open to us we will choose. Decision making is a characteristic implicit within the human makeup. Knowing the consequences of alternatives makes it possible for humans to exercise our responsibilities toward God and other people. In this way, freedom is possible in the midst of controls.

Difficulties arise once certain people acquire an ability to control, manipulate and modify the behavior of others. Such control has always been possible, although increasingly sophisticated techniques open up broader vistas. The critical issue is the goals of the manipulatory techniques. When they aim at enlarging an individual's ability to make decisions, exercise responsibility, relate to fellow beings, find fulfillment in human attributes and respond to God and other people, the techniques have a valuable part to play in promoting God's purposes. They thus uphold the welfare and dignity of beings who are created in God's image. On the other hand, to use manipulatory techniques to further the cause of one group of people over another or even of one individual over another, so that the one will benefit *at the expense* of the other, reduces the techniques to the level of dehumanizing agents. The potentialities of individuals are reduced rather than enhanced; the prospects open to them are narrowed and they become subject—to some degree at least —to the dictates and whims of other individuals. True dialog becomes impossible because the manipulators refuse to be answerable to the manipulated. The equality of individuals as individuals is lost.

Two principles emerge from our considerations. The first is that a society run by an elite class of scientists, capable of technically shaping the environment and people's behavior, is a vision totally opposed to Christian principles. At heart such a vision denies freedom and other features basic to human existence such as love, compassion, concern and justice. Likewise, it refuses to place value on genuine, liberating dialog, thereby reducing men and women to environmentally determined beings who behave well only in response to appropriate rewards.

The second principle is more positive, dealing with behavior *therapy* rather than behavior *management*. In the therapeutic realm, these techniques can be used to overcome learned behavior patterns considered inappropriate or unacceptable. Behavior therapy requires great respect for persons and personal liberty, touching a person's dignity more intimately than the healing of bodily diseases. According to Bernard Häring, "Nobody on this earth should abrogate to himself the *role* of therapist without being invited in freedom, or without intention to be a real partner." These sentiments spring from Häring's Christian view, expressing the reality of human conscience, the power of inner freedom, the decisive value of inner convictions and the capacity to search for ultimate meaning.

Even behavior therapy renders the therapist a social engineer when treatment is sought for conditions that are not directly injurious to the patient. In such cases, when the conditions contravene some social convention, treatment may be required to deal with the social stigma rather than with the conditions per se. Homosexuality may be a prime example. Even when social expectations and human responses are so closely intertwined, however, the needs of the person in his or her wholeness remain paramount.

Psychological conditioning is, as we have seen, subtle and efficient. The possibilities for its misuse are unlimited. The only hope open to us to prevent such misuse and to promote its valuable side is to see others as persons like ourselves. They are not manipulable objects but, like us, have feelings, aspirations, frustrations and hopes. Like us they are people for whom Christ died.

# 6

## Environmental Influences on the Brain

OVER RECENT DECADES it has become increasingly evident that the brain is not isolated from its environment. As we have already seen, brain damage, psychosurgery and psychotropic drugs affect various facets of brain organization. In this chapter we look at some other influences on the brain: malnutrition and the quality of the general sensory environment. Those influences, though more subtle, may tax our value systems to the utmost.

### The Human Face of Malnutrition

Malnutrition is being recognized as almost universally present in today's world. Its influence extends from Appalachia to Ethiopia, from the inner core of our big cities to the rural areas of India and Bangladesh. One of the most significant aspects of malnutrition is that many cases go undetected in the early stages. That is because problems caused by malnutrition cannot be readily recognized as such by ordinary clinical procedures.

The extreme of malnutrition is famine, a frequent occurrence throughout the Middle East and Europe in ancient times. Even this century has witnessed people driven to cannibalism in the face of devastating hunger. In the late 1940s, however, many people were optimistic about winning the battle against hunger. They thought that bumper harvests in the United States and the development of "miracle seeds" would vanquish that dreaded foe and that the densely populated countries of the Third World would attain self-sufficiency in foodstuffs.

History was not so easily overturned. In the 1970s, malnutrition of plague proportions brought on an avalanche of despair. In 1972, for instance, the world's harvest was some 3 per cent short of meeting demands; by 1974, the world's reserves of grain had reached their lowest level for twenty-two years. That was a twenty-six-day supply compared with a supply for ninety-five days in the early 1960s.

At present, it is estimated that half a billion to a billion and a half people suffer from some form of hunger. Of those, about 10,000 die of starvation each week in Africa, Asia and Latin America. The figures vary from year to year, depending on the success of yearly harvests and even on the ambiguity of definitions of *hunger*. When poverty is taken as an indicator, the figures are still enormous. For example, according to a 1977 study published by the National Academy of Sciences, 750 million people in the poorest nations live in extreme poverty, having annual incomes of less than $75. When some of the slightly less poor nations are also taken into account, the figure is increased by several hundreds of millions of individuals. Such figures are beyond our comprehension and tend to leave us numb and unmoved.

We are more likely to be moved by the plight of children. At any given time there are approximately 10 million severely malnourished preschool children, with very many more suffering from moderate forms of malnutrition. All told, about 3 per cent of children under five in low-income countries suffer from severe protein-calorie malnutrition, their body weight being lower than 60 per cent of the standard. Another 80 million preschool children are probably suffering from moderate malnutrition (60-75 per cent of the standard) and 130 to 160 million from mild malnutrition (75-90 per cent of the standard).

Viewed even in that narrow context, malnutrition has enormous social repercussions. It is more accurate to view its occurrence as part of a larger constellation of deprivation. Malnutrition is frequently accompanied by other traits of poverty such as high infant-mortality and prematurity rates and high levels of mental deficiencies. Within that context, the severity of malnutrition appears to be related to such factors as the total number of siblings, number of siblings under the age of two years, family income, food expenditure per person per month, schooling of the mother and father and the likelihood of being the product of an unwanted pregnancy. An additional factor in this constellation of deprivation is illiteracy, which serves to aggravate the other aspects of malnutrition.

In general, one of the contexts of malnutrition is poverty (Fig. 6.1). This, in turn, may be a manifestation of ignorance, adverse climatic conditions, dispossession, urbanization and the economic and commercial structure of the contemporary world. It is in these interrelated contexts that population levels, food production and food consumption need to be viewed.

Stanley Mooneyham, president of World Vision, says: "Poverty is relative but total poverty is absolute, and total poverty is the only term that adequately describes masses of people in the fourth world." Unbelievably, that Fourth World of absolute poverty applies to some 40 per cent of the people living in underdeveloped countries. Included with the Fourth World of hunger are countries such as India, Bangladesh, Pakistan, Ethiopia, Burundi, Chad and Tanzania. In most of these countries, fewer than one person in four is literate; infant mortality rates are as much as ten

*Figure 6.1   The context in which malnutrition has to be viewed. Coexistent with malnutrition is poverty, which itself is the result of the other factors illustrated.*

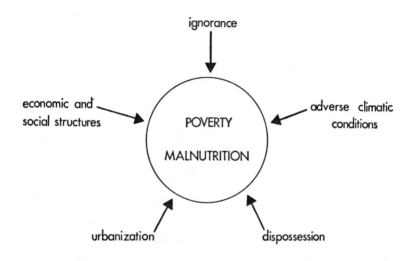

times those in the developed world, and population growth rates are two or three times those in most developed countries (Fig. 6.2). As we shall see, these three features of life have devastating repercussions for the brains and behavior patterns of children and adults in the Fourth World.

Poverty is the pivotal point of more than one vicious circle. In the words of Robert Heilbroner: "It is not just a lack of capital, or just backward ways, or just a population problem or even just a political problem which weighs upon the poorer nations. It is a combination of all these, each aggravating the other. The troubles of underdevelopment feed upon themselves."

Although poverty impinges on the deepest aspirations and expectations of people as individual human beings, the easiest way to express poverty is in financial terms. For example, although the average per capita income in developed Western nations is on the order of $2,400 (in North America

*Figure 6.2   Infant mortality and population growth rates in a range of developed and developing countries.*

| Infant Mortality (deaths in first year of life per 1,000 live births) | | Population growth rate per year (expressed in percentage) | |
|---|---|---|---|
| Sweden | 9 | U.K. | 0.2 |
| U.K. | 16 | West Germany | 0.4 |
| Australia | 17 | U.S.A. | 0.8 |
| U.S.A. | 17 | U.S.S.R. | 0.9 |
| West Germany | 21 | Japan | 1.2 |
| U.S.S.R. | 28 | Canada | 1.4 |
| Chile | 78 | China | 1.4 |
| Guatemala | 81 | Australia | 1.5 |
| Egypt | 100 | India | 2.1 |
| India | 122 | Mozambique | 2.3 |
| Pakistan | 124 | Bangladesh | 2.4 |
| Rwanda | 133 | Ethiopia | 2.6 |
| Malawi | 142 | Nigeria | 2.7 |
| Liberia | 159 | Brazil | 3.0 |
| | | Pakistan | 3.0 |
| | | Mexico | 3.5 |

*Figures in both columns based on U.N. Demographic Year Book, 1975.*

it is well over $4,000), it is only $200 in the underdeveloped world. What is more, this differential is rapidly increasing. These figures tell us something about inequality of wealth at the international level. Yet that is only the beginning of the inequality saga; inequality is even more devastating at the national level. For instance, in Latin America as a whole, 60 per cent of the population have incomes of less than $50 a year and 30 per cent earn up to $190; of the remaining 10 per cent, 9.9 per cent earn over $500, including 0.1 per cent with incomes in excess of $27,000. The inequality of incomes in many Latin American countries increases with the passing of each year.

The plight of many in the underdeveloped countries is appalling. Once poor, they can do little to break out of the vicious poverty cycle. Many years ago, Alfred Marshall said, "The study of the causes of poverty is the study of the causes of degradation of a large part of mankind." His words, true in 1890, are more pressing today as we face growing disparity in the face of growing need.

Poverty, which dominates the underdeveloped nations, brings in its wake ill-health. In some areas 30-50 per cent of all children die before reaching their fifth birthday; in 1970, 36.7 per cent did so in Guinea and 31.0 per cent in Pakistan, as opposed to 1.7 per cent in Sweden. Poverty means that doctors are scarce, particularly in rural areas. Some countries cannot afford to spend more than sixty or seventy cents a year on the health care of each citizen.

Malnutrition, affecting the lives of a majority of human beings today, is one of the most potent forces in our world. In coming years it may even be the major factor in revolutionizing the lifestyles, social values and political systems of both underdeveloped and developed nations.

The term *malnutrition* signifies any form of nutrient imbalance and hence technically includes both undernutrition (too little food) and overnutrition (too much food). We will use malnutrition in its popular sense, restricting it to nutritional deprivation.

Starvation, or extreme undernutrition, leads to a number of well-recognized conditions on the road to death. Wasting of muscles, loss of body fat and wrinkling of skin are manifestations of a general deterioration in which the body, in a desperate attempt to find fuel, is burning up its own body fats, muscles and tissues. A resulting inability to resist infection leads to disease. We shall see that shortage of carbohydrates affects the brain, diminishing a person's ability to comprehend his plight. Deficiency diseases are almost universal in some countries; deficiencies of proteins, vitamin D, thiamin and niacin lead to rickets, beri-beri, pellagra and osteomalacia. Children die from malnutrition-related diseases: gastritis and enteritis, pneumonia and influenza, measles, bronchitis and whooping cough. In 1967 these conditions together accounted for almost 50 per cent of all deaths of children under the age of one year in Ecuador;

in Sweden, they were responsible for less than 4 per cent of these deaths.

The most common deficit is of both proteins and calories. Although it is unwise to separate protein and calorie deficiencies, two syndromes are recognized in severe malnutrition, marasmus and kwashiorkor. In *marasmus,* usually confined to children less than one year old, the principal deficiency is calories. *Kwashiorkor,* by contrast, occurs more frequently in the second year of life and is principally a protein deficiency. There is considerable clinical overlap, marasmus describing a child without edema (excess water) and weighing less than 60 per cent of its expected weight for age and kwashiorkor referring to an edematous child falling within the 60-80 per cent range of weight for age.

One of the most significant points about malnutrition is that many cases are undetected in the early stages. They cannot be readily recognized by ordinary clinical procedures. We are increasingly coming to see that malnutrition is almost universally present in today's world. Its influence extends from Harlem to Ethiopia, from the inner areas of our big cities to the parched rural areas of India and Bangladesh.

## Consequences of Malnutrition for the Brain

As we have seen, malnutrition kills. In Brazil, children under five form less than 20 per cent of the population but account for 80 per cent of all deaths. Malnutrition converts otherwise minor ailments into killers. It leads to prolonged illnesses and chronic infections. It also produces permanent handicaps. Opportunities are lost; education is wasted and a mediocre product of one generation becomes a nonproductive, dependent member of the next. Undernutrition rapidly assumes transgenerational proportions, perpetuating inefficiency, unproductivity and impoverishment.

Malnutrition interferes with a child's motivation as well as with the ability to concentrate and learn. Overall, malnourished children are apathetic and listless, and lack the curiosity essential to normal development. Not surprisingly, they are unable to cope adequately with the demands of schooling. Their mental and physical fatigue as well as frequent bouts of nutrition-related illnesses contribute to poor performance, limited aspirations and a high dropout rate.

The real impact of an economic measure of malnutrition stems from what can (or cannot) be purchased with the available money (Fig. 6.3). With that gap between rich and poor made clear, the biological vulnerability of the poor is exemplified. Figure 6.3 shows that the higher the income in a country, the smaller the percentage of that income spent on food and the greater the percentage of animal protein in the overall dietary protein. Figure 6.4 demonstrates that the richer a country, the greater, by and large, the per capita cereal consumption. One reason for the vast differences in cereal consumption is that Europeans and North Americans eat much of their grain indirectly, that is, through grain-fed livestock and fowl.

Many facets of the grain story are beyond the scope of this brief survey yet are pivotal to the inequality of food availability in poor and rich countries. It is enough to mention that livestock in the rich countries eat as much grain as the combined populations of the two most populous countries,

*Figure 6.3    Allocation of income for food expenditure (mid-1960s).*

| Country | Per capita G.N.P. ($) | Per cent of expenditures allocated to food | Animal protein as per cent of total protein |
|---------|----------------------|-------------------------------------------|---------------------------------------------|
| U.S.A. | 3,980 | 23 | 72 |
| Sweden | 2,620 | 32 | 69 |
| Malaysia | 330 | 49 | 30 |
| Honduras | 260 | 47 | 27 |
| Sri Lanka | 180 | 56 | 18 |
| Ghana | 170 | 64 | 17 |

*Based on U.N. figures issued in 1967 and 1970.*

Figure 6.4 *Per capita cereal consumption in pounds (1972-1974).*

| | |
|---|---|
| U.S.A. | 1850 |
| U.S.S.R. | 1435 |
| European community | 1000 |
| Japan | 620 |
| China | 430 |
| Developing countries (except China) | 395 |

*Based on figures of Economic Research Service, U.S. Department of Agriculture.*

China and India. The food needs of vast numbers in the developing countries, therefore, are tied in complicated ways to the overconsumption and dietary habits of many in the affluent sectors of the world. The knife-edge on which the poor walk is epitomized by Figure 6.3; when some one-half of income is spent on food, little remains for emergency needs, enhancing the environment, or cultural pursuits. The impoverishment of the environment, coupled with poor-quality food, has serious repercussions for the brain and behavior. Further, a general increase in food costs simply cannot be accommodated. Any increase leads to further lowering of nutritional levels, worsening of the all-around environment and yet harsher poverty.

The impact of malnutrition on behavior patterns, intelligence and the brain is a topic of growing concern. The basic fact is that approximately 80 per cent of the growth of the human brain occurs between the end of the second trimester of pregnancy and the end of the second year of life. During that growth spurt, many brain parameters are undergoing rapid change (Fig. 6.5). Any interruption to this growth spurt will, it is argued, affect such processes as the establishment of synaptic connections between nerve cells, the multi-

*Figure 6.5  Components of the growth spurt of the human brain.*

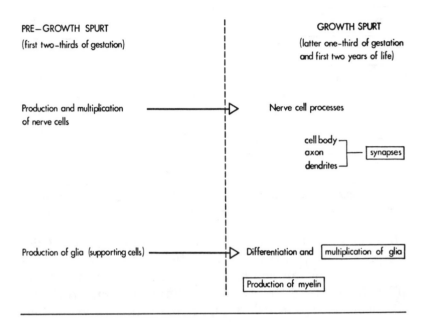

plication of the glia (supporting cells), and the formation of
myelin, the insulating material of the nerve cells. If physical
growth processes occur at specified ages throughout development, it follows that any disruption of that chronological
sequence during the brain's growth spurt will result in long-
term structural and neurological deficits. Even compara-
tively mild nutritional restriction during the period of the
brain's growth spurt may lead to permanent deficits of the
adult brain.

The concept of a vulnerable period of brain development
has a number of implications. It pinpoints the last trimester
of pregnancy and the first two years of postnatal life as a
particularly critical time for human development, and it
suggests that something going even slightly wrong in that
time may have major consequences, which may prove to be
permanent. The evidence on which the idea of nutritional

vulnerability rests comes both from studies on a range of experimental animals and from observations of underprivileged human groups.

As an example of the human studies, consider those carried out by pediatrician Joaquin Cravioto, who, since the early 1960s, has investigated the life and living conditions of the inhabitants of a village of 5,500 people in southwestern Mexico. Cravioto and his co-workers found that schoolchildren who had suffered from severe protein-calorie malnutrition before their thirtieth month of life scored consistently lower in psychological tests compared with equivalent children who had not experienced malnutrition.

In another study, Cravioto looked at the effect of early malnutrition on auditory-visual integration by comparing schoolchildren of shorter stature with their taller companions of the same age. The shorter children showed poorer intersensory development, a factor more closely connected with malnutrition than with environmental influences.

In animal investigations, protein malnutrition inflicted during the brain's growth period has been found to decrease indices such as brain weight, thickness of the cerebral cortex, number of brain cells, amount of brain lipids and hence the extent of formation of myelin, the insulating material around nerves (Fig. 6.6). In addition, evidence suggests a delay in development of some transmitter systems, decrease in synaptic connectivity, and retardation in the maturity of the synaptic junctions themselves.

Under such conditions there is a decrease in thickness of the cerebral cortex. Layering of the cortex may be poorly defined and, as development proceeds, the layers become unduly compressed. Changes in the different cell types within the cortex in malnourished animals are complex, so each component must be assessed independently. For a complete picture of what the malnourished brain is like, we are of course dependent on experimental animals, in particular the rat.

Considerable research interest is currently being shown

*Figure 6.6 Relationship between the brain of an individual and the environment, diet and behavior of that individual. The indices within the central box are of value in determining the development and maturity of the brain.*

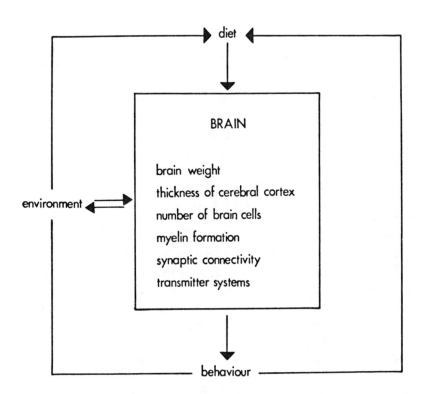

in the synapses between nerve cells. The fact that those tiny areas are affected by malnutrition shows its pervasive influence. The most strategic communication sites of the developing brain are thus exposed to "nutritional insult." In malnourished animals, the number of synapses per nerve cell shows a deficit of around 40 per cent in some nerve terminals. Further, the remaining synapses are structurally and probably functionally modified as well. The size of the synapses and even the number and size of the synaptic vesicles are diminished in the brains of malnourished animals. The important thickenings at the synaptic junction are not as wide, and the curvature of the junction is altered, suggesting that fundamental changes have occurred in the neurotransmitter systems. Overall, the development of synaptic junctions is delayed by malnutrition.

Is it possible subsequently to rectify such deficits? Experimental evidence on rehabilitation is sparse and confused, but suggests that only a limited amount of "catch-up" takes place when the diet is made adequate. Any distinction between "retarded" brain development and "abnormal" development is tenuous. The final measures of brain parameters in nutritionally rehabilitated animals seem to fall midway between those for well-nourished and malnourished ones.

Evidence for catch-up among human groups is also conflicting. For example, Cravioto and associates, in a study of twenty children undergoing nutritional rehabilitation after severe protein-calorie malnutrition, concluded that children over fifteen months of age at the time of the malnutrition showed improvement over a six-month period. By contrast, children less than six months of age may be permanently affected. One must be careful, however, because the apathy and unresponsiveness of severely protein-malnourished children leads to the critical stages of cognition being missed. Stages of brain development do not occur because essential experiences have not occurred. Other environmental factors of potential significance include the effects of hospitalization and any decreased response of the mother to an unresponsive child.

By contrast, two American nutritionists, H. P. Chase and H. P. Martin, in a study of children suffering from undernutrition during the first four months of life and later nutritionally rehabilitated, came to a more optimistic conclusion. According to their data, those children three years later had developmental quotients equal to those of control children.

What can we conclude, at present, from such investigations? There can be little doubt that malnutrition itself is one factor, along with environmental and social factors, depressing the cognitive development of previously malnourished children (Fig. 6.6). The relative contributions of the factors is still open to debate. It should be kept in mind, though, that malnourished infants almost invariably are also exposed to poor housing, low levels of educational achievement, high infection rates and all sorts of taboos.

It has been suggested, but not proven, that permanent intellectual deficit occurs in malnourished children only where the nonnutritional environment is also poor. That suggestion has some support from animal investigations. Whatever its validity, it reiterates the overall interdependence of components of human growth.

Cravioto, aware that malnutrition does not occur independently, wanted to find what associations exist between malnutrition and various aspects of a child's environment. He compared such things as the parents' height, age and weight, their personal cleanliness, literacy and educational level, the frequency with which they read newspapers and the proportion of their annual income spent on food. None showed any significant association with the presence or absence in the family of malnourished children. But a positive finding emerged when he examined the mothers' radio-listening habits. The mothers of severely malnourished children in Cravioto's Mexican village listened much less frequently to the radio than did those of healthier children. That finding shows one facet of a relationship now being recognized: general environmental stimulation, which is usually stimulation in the home, protects a child against the worst effects of malnutrition. More generally, the factors precipitating malnutrition in a home are similar to the factors responsible for minimal stimulation in that home. In other words, malnutrition primarily occurs within environments in which many other forces may also limit the individual's development.

We are living not in "one world" but in at least two

worlds: the world of the rich and the world of the poor, the haves and the have-nots; the world of need and the world of plenty, the hungry and the full. Consider a few comparisons. In England and Wales there is one doctor for 900 people; the ratio in rural Kenya is one for 50,000. In rural Senegal in 1960 the death rate of children aged two to five years was forty times higher than in France. A teen-ager in Tanzania has about one per cent of the educational opportunities of a teen-ager in North America. The G.N.P. (gross national product) per person in Malawi is approximately one-fiftieth that in Sweden. And so on and on. The best summary, perhaps, is seen in the life expectancy in different countries, varying between more than seventy years in most rich countries to as little as twenty-five years in some poor countries.

Inequality of wealth is the foundation on which the inequality of malnutrition has been built. Malnutrition has devastating effects on lifestyles and aspirations: nutrition is central to determining what we are as human beings. Poor people are not just poor; they are impoverished as human beings. In that sense, poverty can be defined as a condition that restricts the development of human creativity and resourcefulness. Here again, we see two worlds: a poor world with its cultural impoverishment and a rich world with opportunities for cultural enrichment and control of the environment. The people in those worlds have become different kinds of people: some have hope as human beings and others have little or no hope. The horizons of the majority of people in our world are limited by their need to acquire food to stave off the next death in the family.

## The Brain's Environment

The possibility that experiential changes have neurological consequences has long been recognized, with research dating back to the 1780s. More recently Santiago Ramón y Cajal, Donald Hebb and Sir John Eccles have, in different ways, suggested that information derived from experience

Figure 6.7 *The three environments employed to test the effects of differential environments on the brain and behavior of rats: a. social condition; b. impoverished condition; c. enriched condition. From "Brain Changes in Response to Experience." Copyright © 1972 by Scientific American, Inc. All rights reserved.*

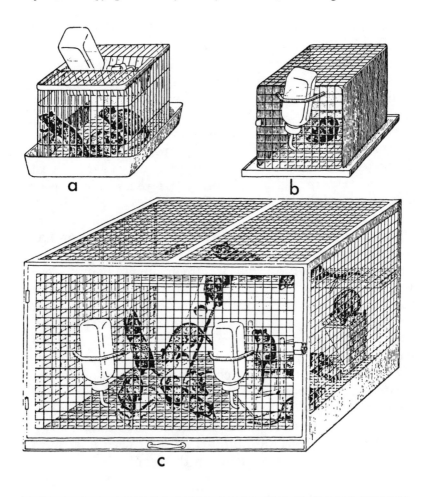

may bring about behavioral changes in animals by modifying synaptic connections within the brain.

Decisive work in this realm has been done by psychologist Mark Rosenzweig and his colleagues at the University of

Calfornia in Berkeley. In conjunction with biochemist Edward Bennett and anatomist Marian Diamond, they began in the early 1960s to subject rats to different living conditions. These have generally been of the three types illustrated in Figure 6.7. In the impoverished condition (IC), a single rat lives undisturbed in a small cage, lacking toys of any sort. In the social condition (SC), three rats live together in a larger cage, but still without toys. At the upper end of the continuum is the enriched condition (EC), with nine or ten rats living together in a very large cage, equipped with ample toys which are changed every day.

In most of the experiments to date, rats have been placed in the cages at weaning when they are 25 days old and left in them for periods of up to 160 days. Maximum effects on the rats' brains are obtained after 30 days of differential experience (Fig. 6.8), although differences in brain structure have been seen after as little as 4 days. The brain differences persist for as long as the different environments persist. Longer periods of separate rearing, however, are associated with smaller brain differences, while the older an animal is

*Figure 6.8  Rats placed in an enriched environment (EC) at 25 days of age, and kept there for 30 days, have brains that differ in certain respects from rats placed in an impoverished environment (IC) for the same time period.*

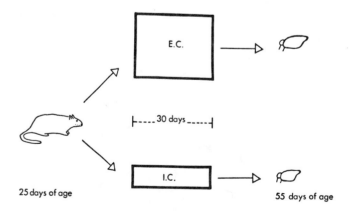

when the differential rearing is commenced, the smaller are the observed differences.

Some rats have been reared from weaning in IC or EC environments, then switched to the opposite environment for an equal period of time (Fig. 6.9). With that type of arrangement it has been found that an enriched environment in the second period (30 days) appears to overcome the effects of deprivation during the first period (30 days). Perhaps even more interesting is the finding that an enriched environment during the first 30 days affords some protection against the effects of a subsequently impoverished environment. With longer periods of time, the secondary environment assumes a major role in the final outcome of the brain; prolonged exposure to a secondary environment (whether enriched or impoverished) modifies and may even nullify the effects of the primary environment.

Some of Rosenzweig's results can be said to be due to the the effects of impoverishment, others to the predominant role of enrichment. If the animals in the standard social con-

*Figure 6.9 Switchover experiments in which rats are first placed in an enriched environment (EC) and subsequently transferred to an impoverished environment (IC) or vice versa.*

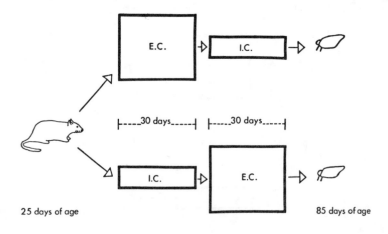

dition thus constitute a neutral baseline, one is essentially saying that brain parameters can be "improved" by a particularly favorable environment (Fig. 6.10a). The social repercussions of this issue affect the manner in which the data are applied to the human situation.

After all, if the brains of most people can be "improved" by contact with a more stimulating environment, leading to more intelligent and creative individuals, a strong case for advocating such environments at all stages of people's lives can be made. Conversely, if the enriched environmental condition represents the genetic upper limit to an individual's potential, any differences between the enriched and impoverished conditions reflect the extent to which normal development has been retarded by sensory deprivation (Fig. 6.10b). If that is true, it would be legitimate to speak only about impoverishment as the factor creating the environmental differences.

Evidence favoring either alternative possibility is sketchy at present. What can be said with certainty is that those children reared in an unexciting and unstimulating environment are being deprived biologically as well as socially. They will not attain anything approaching their full development. Exactly the same situation applies to adults, who can suffer impoverishment as adults in addition to whatever deficits remain from childhood. One would also like to think that improvement can be attained by making the environment more stimulating. This is probably so, although one must be careful to define terms precisely. It would be unrealistic to expect to make up huge deficits, particularly well into adult life. Nevertheless, the brain is an infinitely more malleable piece of equipment than once was imagined, both for good and ill, and the quality of the environment in which people live is always of immense importance.

What specific measurements constitute the evidence in favor of sensory environmental effects on the brain? As with the malnutrition studies, the data range from rather gross

*Figure 6.10 Diagram illustrating the alternative concepts of regarding a. the standard environment (SC) and b. the enriched environment (EC) as the respective baselines for considering the quality of the environment.*

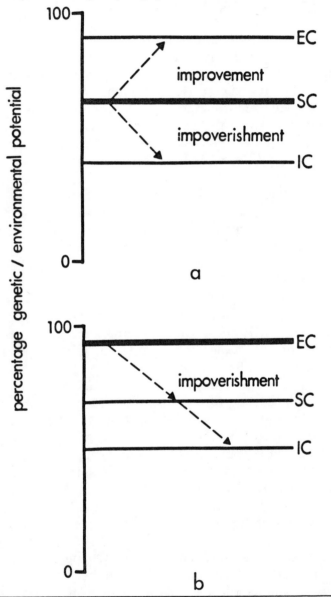

ones such as brain weight and size to highly specific ones such as the number and size of nerve cells and even the number and size of synapses (Fig. 1.15 and 1.16). In between these extremes, the thickness of the cerebral cortex and the extent of dendritic branching have also been examined. In general terms the brains from rats living in enriched environments are heavier, have deeper cortices, larger nerve cells with longer and more complex branching dendrites, and larger but less numerous synapses. At the biochemical level, protein changes have been found in the brains of enriched rats, while various modifications to enzymes involved in neurotransmission have also been recorded.

How do the animals subjected to different environments actually behave? Of the many tests of behavioral ability administered, it is maze-learning that brings to the fore the consistently superior performance of the enriched-environment animals. Certain other tests, such as discrimination-reversal learning, point in the same direction. With both structural and behavioral parameters, however, effects vary. Some parts of the brain appear to be more susceptible to environmental variation than others, and animals react more at certain ages than at others.

## Malnutrition in a Wider Environment

As noted earlier, malnutrition occurs as part of a much wider context of poverty and general deprivation. The context outlined in Figure 6.1 amounts to a condition of impoverishment and lack of well-being. Every aspect of the environment of a malnourished person will be found to be drab and depressing, lacking the elements essential for lively, stimulating surroundings. With existence reduced to the meanest physical levels, there is neither time nor energy for broadening interests or developing cultural horizons. In short, such an existence, even in the presence of barely adequate food, resembles the impoverished environment of an isolated rat in its small cage.

In communities in which malnutrition is endemic there is

a close interplay between the nutritional deprivation and general environmental impoverishment. The two can hardly be separated as causal factors for the retarded brain development and behavioral consequences seen in individuals. The compounding of deficiencies found in such deprived individuals leads to an air of gloom. If nothing can be done to alleviate one's plight, why bother? Indeed, doing research in such areas has even been questioned on the grounds that research can only confirm whatever gloomy predictions are current.

Without minimizing the known effects of malnutrition and environmental deprivation on the brains and hence personalities of individuals affected in early life, such pessimistic catastrophism needs to be challenged. Although brain growth is retarded by malnutrition during early development, some catch-up does appear to be possible later on if good nutrition is available. And it now appears likely that social stimulation can, at least to a limited degree, offset the ill effects of poor nutrition. Some of the possibilities are depicted in Figure 6.11.

A child's ultimate intellectual status is the end result of interaction between nutrition and other environmental factors such as social stimulation. Stimulation and optimal nutrition must both be viewed as answers to the threat of poverty. In one series of animal experiments it was noticed that malnutrition increases the contact time between a mother rat and her suckling pups, reducing the amount of time the pups are free to explore their surroundings. The same situation has been noted for human mother-infant interactions. Malnutrition thus leads to less social stimulation, doubly affecting the deprived young. Both forms of deprivation lead to intellectual impairment and reduction in learning capacity (Fig. 6.11).

The optimistic side of that interaction is that the behavioral deficits in malnourished animals are considerably reduced by a period of rearing under very enriched conditions. This work is in its infancy, and yet it fits in with the

Figure 6.11 *Interrelationship between (a) early malnutrition, environmental deprivation and brain impairment, and (b) optimal nutrition, optimal environmental stimulation and whatever catch-up is possible in brain function following initial impairment.*

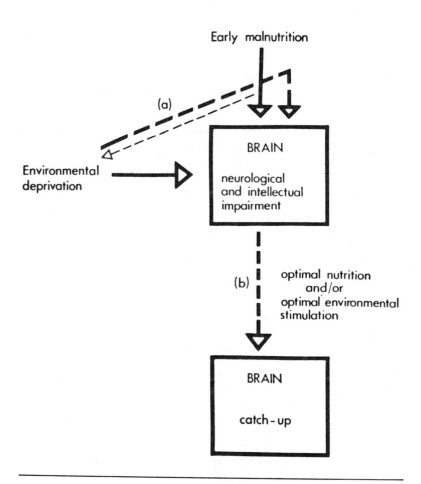

results of other studies showing that animals with brain lesions perform better on behavioral tests if exposed to enriched environments either before or after the lesion is inflicted. The beneficial effects of environmental enrichment on behavioral recovery evidently extend to some structural indices in the brains. One hopes that for humans also a greater degree of recovery from brain damage can occur when the individual is exposed to an enriched, stimulating environment than when left to idle in a drab, quiet and colorless world.

One cannot be dogmatic on this issue in the human realm because conflicting reports on different groups of children abound. One of the most clear-cut studies concerns a group of Korean orphans who, in the late 1950s and '60s, were adopted during early life (average age eighteen) by U.S. parents. The children's environment underwent a radical change. They were divided for comparison into three groups: malnourished, moderately nourished and well nourished. When tested in the early 1970s, all three groups surpassed the expected mean for Korean children in both height and weight, although below the 50th percentile on an American standard. All the groups reached or exceeded mean IQ values of American children. What is striking is that even the severely malnourished children surpassed Korean norms of height and weight, and the marked initial size differences between the malnourished and well-nourished infants greatly decreased.

Severe early malnutrition of prolonged duration produces brain and behavioral deficits which cannot be eradicated. Nevertheless, rehabilitation in the form of optimal nutrition and a stimulating, demanding environment, can in all probability diminish those deficits. The absence of rehabilitation, however, insures that the disadvantaged children will become disadvantaged adults who in their turn will produce further disadvantaged children in a recurring cycle of debilitation.

### Inequality and Human Responsibility

The lives and prospects of *people*, not just isolated brains or detached synapses, are placed in peril by poverty. People as people must be uppermost in our thinking, and with them the environments in which they find themselves. Even in a book on the brain, we cannot completely overlook the subject of the quality of our environment. Since what is good for people is frequently also good for the environment, many facets of a debate about people apply equally to the environmental debate.

Debate in both of these areas owes much to Christian thought-forms, so these shall be used in formulating relevant guidelines.

The fundamental principle is that of God's creation: all that exists owes its being to the thought and action of God. What is more, the creation was initially deemed *very good* by God himself. The human race was included within that characterization, from which we may conclude that God was pleased with humanity, with the original environment as a whole and with the interrelationship of the two. All these aspects of the creation are therefore important to God and derive meaning and significance from that importance. In spite of the Fall, the "very good" designation of man and the environment still holds, although both are now tarnished by self-centeredness, greed and rebellion against God's authority.

That assertion is substantiated by the *Incarnation*, in which God so demonstrated his regard and concern for the created world, and for humanity that he took to himself human identity. In so doing he implicitly pronounced a verdict of very, very good upon mankind, thereby stressing our significance and need of redemption. The Incarnation is the epitome of God's identification with the created order, bestowing on it—even in its fallen state—a grandeur and value of eternal dimensions. Nothing in creation is to be despised, although that principle requires some detailed working out. The human creation in the image and after the likeness of God must be taken into account.

Two divergent aspects characterize human beings, namely, their transcendence and immanence—or more accurately, their relative transcendence and their immanence. In them we see, on the one hand, the manner in which we reflect important features of God's own character and, on the other, our dependence on our biological environment. Consideration of both facets brings out the responsibility that must be exercised by people in privileged societies, and the damage that can be inflicted on people exposed to malnutrition and impoverished environments. Those of us living in the affluent sector of our world have a responsibility to work out what our privileges might mean in a world ordered and cared for by God.

All human beings have intrinsic dignity because of who they are, a dignity bestowed on them by God in both creation and redemption. Dignity deriving from God is an integral feature of what humans *are,* rather than of what they can *do.* Human dignity is an ever present facet of human existence and applies equally to all individuals, regardless of their political, social or nutritional status. Their dignity is irrespective of their worth according to the criteria of particular social systems. Even those teetering on the brink of starvation, with no functional value in society, have, in Professor Helmut Thielicke's phrase, an "alien dignity"—a dignity according to God's criteria even if alien according to human assessment. The Lausanne Covenant expressed that sentiment in these words: "Because mankind is made in the image of God, every person... has an intrinsic dignity because of which he should be respected and served, not exploited...."

God is concerned with people regardless of their superficial characteristics. Further, God is concerned with justice and compassion in human society. That concern was eloquently and movingly brought out by the Old Testament prophet Amos when he stressed the importance of human rights, freedom, compassion and individual integrity.

The relationship of human beings to their Creator thus implies or includes a responsibility to their neighbors. Because people were created to live in community, the manner in which we live out our interpersonal relationships is important in God's sight. Relationships between groups of individuals are also important.

As John Stott phrases it, "God created man, who is my neighbour, a body-soul-in-community." He continues, "If we love our neighbour as God made him, we must inevitably be concerned for his total welfare, the good of his soul, his body and his community." The reason we should be concerned for the social welfare of others is the compassion of Christ himself.

How to apply these principles of wholeness to malnourished people is obvious. They are our responsibility because they are not only our neighbors, they are underprivileged. We are responsible for them on both counts. God's concern for the hungry rings out time and again through the pages of Scripture. For instance, in Isaiah 58:6-10, we read: "Is not this what I require of you as a fast . . .? Is it not sharing your food with the hungry, taking the homeless poor into your house . . .? If you feed the hungry from your own plenty and satisfy the needs of the wretched, then your light will rise like dawn out of darkness. . . ." Again in Psalm 146:7 we are reminded that "The LORD feeds the hungry and sets the prisoner free." Moreover, in Proverbs 25:21 we are exhorted to give bread to our enemy when he is hungry and water when he is thirsty. In Ezekiel 18:7 one of the marks of the righteous is that they give bread to the hungry. The New Testament has many injunctions relating to the poor, the needy and the hungry. Mary, extolling the wonderful works of God, exclaimed: "The hungry he has satisfied with good things, the rich [he has] sent empty away" (Lk. 1:53).

God's general concern for the poor is clear. Some writers argue that God actually identifies with the poor. Ronald Sider writes: "God not only acts in history to liberate the poor, but in a mysterious way that we can only half fathom, the Sovereign of the universe identifies with the weak and destitute."

The Christian response to the deprived and underprivileged of the world should be one of love, viewing them as people of dignity having worth equal to our own. We should treat them in a manner commensurate with their status in God's sight. Further, justice and righteousness are demanded of us. The Israelites among whom the prophet Amos lived were very religious, although their religion was far from pure and made little difference in their social attitudes. Perhaps it is significant that their social misdemeanors were the first reason quoted by Amos for God's displeasure.

God's concern for social justice is so great that his people should put justice above everything else within society. The Israelites turned justice upside-down, according to Amos, bringing righteousness to the ground. The link between justice and righteousness demonstrates the interrelatedness of social and religious ideals.

Much earlier in Jewish history the concept of social justice was unequivocally written into their way of life. Among God's rules about conduct, the Jews were instructed thus: "You shall not pervert justice, either by favouring the poor or by subservience to the great. You shall judge your fellow-countryman with strict justice" (Lev. 19:15). Integrity was thus closely linked to the "neighbor" concept. A person must be treated as a human being, which entails scrupulous justice.

Justice is not an abstract concept to be viewed idealistically. It is a basic ingredient of equitable societies and of an equitable world. If societies are not equitable, justice is at a premium simply because lack of justice is closely associated with greed, an association that surfaces repeatedly in the Old Testament. People who are committed to justice must build justice into their social structures.

Christ came to demonstrate the reality and nature of justice, since nothing less is consonant with either human dignity or the character of God. The right of all people to be treated as individuals of value should also lead us to realize that individuals are of greater value than possessions. People are so much more important than things that the life of even the most degraded person should be worth more than the costliest possessions. We who are affluent cannot escape our obligation to work toward a society in which the worst consequences of malnutrition and environmental deprivation are at least minimized. Malnutrition is not merely a biological problem; it is a moral problem, a social problem and a political problem.

# 7

## The New Consciousness

ONE OF THE PERENNIAL characteristics of the human race is its desire to go beyond what is already known. That desire has led to a panaply of great human achievements. Human beings seem to have an insatiable longing to extend themselves and their powers in scientific, artistic, athletic and cultural realms. Such feats are just one side of the coin, however. The other side is the concern of human beings to transcend, not simply their previous achievements, but their own physical presence.

### Transcending the Physical
To transcend the physical is an expression of religious concern. Yet emphasis is often placed on human destiny as viewed from man's perspective rather than God's. Biofeedback, Transcendental Meditation, yoga therapy, holistic medicine, magical forms of faith healing, parapsychology and sorcery are all, to some extent, efforts toward transcendence.

Some of those pursuits are truly ancient, but new emphases have emerged of late to give some of them a semblance of scientific respectability. For instance, Marilyn Ferguson, in her influential book *The Brain Revolution,* has written: "There is an enormous groundswell of scientific interest in practices considered quackery a brief decade ago, in altered states of consciousness, unorthodox healing, and parapsychology." That interest has been especially pronounced in the relationship between mind and body, and particularly in ways in which the mind might achieve preeminence over the body.

Meditators, in particular Zen and yoga meditators, have long been concerned with this domain. Until very recent years, however, the alleged feats of such meditators were treated with the utmost caution, and often with outright skepticism, by Western scientists. Such phenomenal control of the body by the mind had not been convincingly demonstrated in adequately controlled scientific studies, and no established concepts of the mind-body relationship led one to expect the mind to be more powerful than the body. Many Western scientists were skeptical even about the existence of the mind as an entity worthy of serious discussion.

The distinction between well-established nutritional, pharmacological and surgical approaches to the brain and unorthodox approaches such as meditation is an immense one. The distinction is between approaches which are the product of science and technology and others which are independent of science and technology. In a sense the two types of approach are mutually exclusive, with emphasis in Western science on the objective, impersonal approach and in Eastern mysticism on the intuitive, subjective approach.

That simple dichotomy has undergone a major upheaval with the advent of biofeedback and, in its wake, a renewed interest in the West on meditation. According to Barbara Brown, in her book *New Mind, New Body:* "Biofeedback and biofeedback training attracted more scientists . . . and everyone was dreaming of a way to control the uncontrollable inner man, a way to know the self, a way to prevent or cure illnesses, a way to make the mind more mindly, a way perhaps to genius.... Suddenly, out of nowhere had come the lost thread between mind and body, the resurgence of a buried memory as ancient as man himself. There was indeed more to man than the physical self."

Many people have always believed that the physical can be influenced, perhaps transcended, by the mind. One might say that the reality of that phenomenon is beginning to permeate the thinking of Westerners in spite of their long-standing dependence on scientific and analytical approaches to reality. In Western academic circles it has frequently been asserted that there is no longer any room for religious answers. That assertion is being challenged by a plethora of consciousness-changing techniques and a counterassertion that there is no longer any place for the objective. The framework of much Western thinking is under attack by beliefs and attitudes owing much to Eastern mystical traditions, yet apparently at home amid the turmoil, upheaval and uncertainty of contemporary Western society. Some would describe these trends as constituting a global synthesis: Eastern mysticism is being utilized as a means of humanizing Western technology.

There can be no doubt that, in response to widespread feelings of alienation, depersonalization and dehumanization in Western technological societies, a major *consciousness movement* has arisen. It has directly challenged certain oppressive assumptions of technocratic Western society. It has not been afraid to charge rationalist and materialist culture with depleting the quality of human life. According to David Fetcho, a former editor of *Spiritual Counterfeits Project Journal,* Eastern metaphysics and the "new consciousness" assert that our normal way of looking at things is deficient, frequently programmed by the greed conditioned into us by television advertising.

The consciousness movement is a highly syncretistic

and eclectic compendium of techniques ranging from yoga to self-awareness. Nevertheless, common to all of them is a longing to transcend ordinary consciousness and so discover some higher power within the individual. Inherent within that longing is a notion of *altered states of consciousness,* based on the belief that our ordinary, everyday conscious-ness is subjective, arbitrary and culturally determined. That belief leads one to accept as equally real and coherent quite different ways of perceiving the world and organizing one's activities within it.

Charles Tart, a professor of psychology at the University of California at Davis, is a leader of the movement into scientific exploration of "altered states of consciousness," having edited a book with that title back in 1969. He now prefers the term *"discrete* states of consciousness" which he

*Figure 7.1 Diagrammatic representation of discrete states of consciousness, showing the way in which different states can be distinguished on the basis of vari-ations in degree of rationality and ability to hallucinate. Reprinted, with modifica-tions, from J. C. Brash, ed.,* Cunningham's Textbook of Anatomy. *Used by permis-sion of Oxford University Press.*

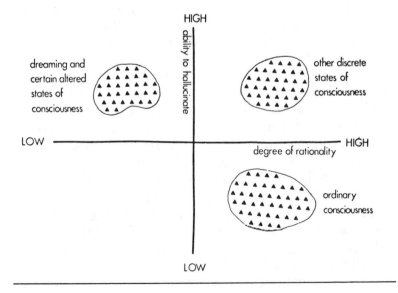

uses to describe radical changes in the organization of consciousness; such changes are reflected in the terms *awake, dreaming, hypnotized* and *meditative.* For instance, as depicted in Figure 7.1, ordinary consciousness is characterized by a high degree of rationality and a low degree of hallucinatory ability. People vary in these two abilities and there are limitations on both within the domain of ordinary consciousness. By contrast, dreaming is characterized by a high degree of imagination and a relatively small amount of rationality. The third state illustrated in Figure 7.1 is another form of dreaming with degrees of rationality and imagination quite different from ordinary dreaming.

Discrete states of consciousness as envisaged by Tart deal with what we may consider normal experience. By contrast, discrete *altered* states of consciousness refer to a discrete state of consciousness different from some baseline state of consciousness. It requires, to use Tart's expression, a "quantum jump" to another region of experiential space, possibly by the use of psychedelic drugs or certain mystical regimens. The intention is to tap and amplify latent human potentials for personal and cultural development.

Basic to Tart's approach is the view that our ordinary state of consciousness is, at best, a semiarbitrary one. He claims that cultural biases are built into our consciousness. The science we are familiar with is an ordinary state-of-consciousness science and hence it too is in many respects culture-bound. Tart claims to foresee the possibility of structuring a totally different type of science within a discrete altered state of consciousness. Such a science would entail radically different ways of organizing our observations and conceptualizations of the universe.

For Charles Tart, as for others in the new-consciousness movement, there is an intimate interaction between beliefs and perceptions. Their emphasis on the limitations and arbitrary nature of ordinary consciousness leads them to a commitment to transcend those limits by organizing their minds along other lines. Hence they are fascinated with the use of psychedelic drugs, meditation, the practice of yoga and various other spiritual disciplines stemming from Eastern mystical traditions.

Another psychologist prominent in the new-consciousness movement is Robert Ornstein of the Langley Porter Neuropsychiatric Institute at the University of California. Ornstein contends that two major modes of consciousness are available, one *analytical,* the other *holistic.* The analytical mode is linear and rational; the holistic is arational and intuitive. Like Tart, Ornstein seeks to pinpoint the limitations of ordinary consciousness. Stressing the degree to which consciousness is a personal construction adapted for our survival, he sees it as analytical and object-centered. It separates us from other objects and organisms. The logic of Ornstein's argument leads him, like Tart, to the conclusion that, if ordinary consciousness is a personal construction, other constructions and other consciousnesses are potentially available to us.

Unlike Tart, however, Ornstein is an advocate neither of the concept of numerous discrete states of consciousness nor of the lasting value of psychedelic drugs in bringing about a radical disruption of normal consciousness. He is more concerned with the esoteric (mystical) psychologies, which "approach psychology as a practical, personal discipline and emphasize techniques that effect alterations in body states and in consciousness for the purpose of gathering knowledge that is other than, but additional to, the intellectual."

Ornstein quotes with approval the physiological self-mastery, the influence of body states on consciousness and the concept of subtle body energies inherent within the esoteric traditions exemplified by yoga, Zen and Sufism. Two additional characteristics of these traditions are nonattachment and the inhibition of thought. With regard to the latter a function of concentrative meditation is to turn off the active verbal mode and to place ordinary thoughts in abeyance for a while. The aim is to rid the practitioner of a strict reliance on verbal intellectuality. In a similar vein, nonattachment is designed to destructure normal consciousness and aims at present-centeredness. It is part of a shift from the individual, analytical consciousness to a mode that depends on training the intuitive side of our makeup, with the overall perspective of holism rather than individuality. The esoteric traditions emphasize body movement, music, spatial forms, sounds, crafts and dreams, rather than a rational approach to reality.

"The new consciousness," to quote James Sire in his book *The Universe Next Door,* "is a world view whose time has come." For an increasing number of Western thinkers it is a foundation for hope. They are taking a quantum leap into a new way of being; they are evolving into a new (and, by definition, better) species; they are moving toward full health and liberating creativity; they are creeping out of the cavern of the old consciousness and into the full dawn of the potential offered by the new consciousness. For some, a true understanding of consciousness is the key that will unlock absolute power over reality. Not surprisingly, therefore, many see humanity as on the brink of a new understanding of itself and its world, an understanding based on this new philosophy and conception of consciousness.

Since the philosophical issues raised by the new consciousness stem in part from our lack of understanding of the brain, they are relevant for a book on the brain. It is true that technology has revolutionized our understanding of the bodily organ that makes us human, and in so doing has exposed the human brain to perilous assaults on its integrity. Yet we barely comprehend what makes the brain the seat of consciousness, self-awareness, self-reflection, motivation and creativity.

Ironically, one finds exactly opposite evaluations of the state of present accomplishments. To some, the efficiency of brain technology is so frightening as to produce an antitechnological backlash. To others, brain technology is so inefficient that it has become the playground of charlatans.

The task of evaluating the merits of unorthodox brain research is formidable. Not long ago the feats of yoga and Zen masters were generally dismissed as clever fraud. Today some of their feats find acceptance in the realm of biofeedback, which itself occupies a position on the edge of orthodoxy. Meditation, once the preserve of the East but now a legitimate study for Western psychologists, is beginning to take its place among the armamentarium of medico-technological tools.

The major difficulty is that once mind and brain are separated, once the mind is granted complete autonomy, the way is open to all kinds of nonobjective beliefs parading before us in the name of science. The new-consciousness frontier, an exciting adventure for some, must not be prejudged without careful study; nevertheless it is a haven for untested, unprovable and facetious hypotheses. In humanity's desperation to escape the bondage of technology, we must be wary of entering a new bondage.

We find ourselves walking a tightrope. If we overbalance on one side we descend into reductionism, the child of technology, with the brain reduced to a pathetic collection of nerve cells and with human beings transformed into machines. If we overbalance on the other side we drop into a subjective and irrational world of relative consciousness phenomena, in which everything is possible but little can be substantiated. Retaining our balance leads to a future with fresh concepts and new categories, even surprises perhaps, but undoubtedly with any essential technological expertise under the control of the human brain.

### Biofeedback

It has been known for centuries that yogis are capable of controlling autonomic or involuntary nervous functions such as heart and respiratory rates. Claims have been made that some are capable of voluntarily stopping their heartbeat or of surviving for extended periods in an "airtight" pit. Investigations of such phenomena in the 1930s and '50s led to conflicting results. Most reputable scientists were skeptical about the feasibility of consciously controlling any involuntary functions.

In the late 1960s, however, Neal Miller and a group of psychologists announced that they had trained rats to alter visceral activities such as heart rate, intestinal motility and urinary output by the technique known as operant conditioning. Working on the premise that, as Miller wryly puts it, humans "in this respect are as smart as rats," Miller and other researchers trained humans to raise and lower their blood pressures and hand temperatures, using instruments to monitor their performance. Such studies led to the biofeedback revolution, which in the minds of some promises cures for all kinds of illnesses as well as bliss-on-demand for the mystically inclined.

Biofeedback is a term given to a set of techniques used in the investigation of learned self-control of physiological activity. It includes the use of instrumentation to mirror psychophysical processes of which the individual is not normally aware, and then to bring those processes under voluntary control. In order to accomplish that, the individual must be given immediate information about the physiological state in question—muscle tension, brainwave activity, heart rate and so on. With such "feedback," the individual can become a more active participant in the regulation of bodily functions. Since these physiological events are related to specific psychological states, individuals learn to control their mental states and especially their emotions. Biofeedback is, therefore, a method of changing consciousness.

Biofeedback has concentrated on three principal areas: the heart, muscles and brain. All three will be touched on here, with emphasis on the brain effects.

One of the yogis alleged to be capable of stopping his heart for twenty seconds or so is Swami Rama. Physiological investigations on him have demonstrated not only that feat but also his ability to alter the temperature of the two sides of the palm of one hand in different directions. Experimentation in the West in the 1960s suggested that the heart rate of volunteers could be controlled if a reward was provided. The reward for changing heart rate was simply the satisfaction of hearing or seeing a monitor of the altered heart rate.

The most influential series of studies on experimental animals has been carried out by Neal Miller and co-workers at Rockefeller University. Miller set out to prove that autonomic (involuntary) functions, such as heart rate, can be made to respond to an external signal without using the stimulus that normally evokes the response. The difficulty confronting him was that the visceral responses easiest to measure—heart rate, vasomotor responses and the galvanic skin response—are all affected by skeletal responses from activities such as exercise, breathing and the contraction of muscles. To overcome that difficulty, he adopted the ingenious method of paralyzing all muscles of the body by administration of the drug curare. Since "reward" was an integral part of the biofeedback study, a way had to be devised to tell the heart that it had correctly performed its task of slowing down or speeding up. That obstacle was overcome by directly stimulating the rewarding areas of the brain.

Using that complex experimental system it was found that rats rewarded for an increase in heart rate showed a statistically reliable increase, and rats rewarded for a decrease showed a statistically reliable decrease. Experiments on intestinal contractions showed similar results. Later it was demonstrated that rates of urine formation and of blood flow to the stomach can be modified using the same techniques. Changes in blood pressure can also be learned. Rats rewarded for increases in blood pressure showed further increases; those rewarded for decreases showed decreases. Such changes appear to be independent of heart rate and temperature changes.

Before exploring the implications of these results for humans, one other piece of information obtained by Miller's group should be mentioned. Rather unexpectedly the experimenters noted that, after learning to alter their heart rate, the rats demonstrated general emotional effects. Rats which had been rewarded for decreasing their heart rate learned well, whereas those rewarded for increasing their heart rate did not learn as well. It was concluded that the rats whose heart rates had increased also showed an increase in emotionality.

Enthusiastic advocates of biofeedback procedures have quickly grasped the potential significance of the rat studies. They argue that the possibilities of psychosomatic *health* should be investigated, on the assumption that the mind can be as effective in *relieving* illnesses as in causing them. The mind-body relationship and the mind's capabilities are the focus of Elmer and Alyce Green at the Psychophysical Research Laboratory of the Menninger Foundation in Topeka, Kansas. The Greens assert that it is possible to change wrong stress-reactions by learning mental control. If so, biofeedback should have important therapeutic uses.

Clinical studies of biofeedback training are still confusing, however. Initial claims have generally not been borne out in clinical practice. Heart-rate studies may be useful in control of cardiac arrhythmias, but few controlled investigations have been carried out. That form of biofeedback should have practical application in the management of anxiety about the heart. Although blood-pressure biofeedback appears to be capable of decreasing blood pressure in hypertensive (high blood pressure) patients by about fifteen millimeters of mercury, it is unclear whether feedback training is more effective in that regard than simple relaxation. Two other forms of biofeedback, namely, skin temperature and electrodermal feedback, are both said to be valuable in the treatment of hypertension. Other conditions amenable to skin temperature training are migraine and asthma. Electrodermal feedback, using the galvanic skin response (GSR), is claimed to be of value in treating phobias and anxiety reactions as well as conditions such as asthma and stuttering.

Biofeedback has been utilized in the control of muscles

and single muscle units. Some of the most impressive results of biofeedback procedures have been obtained using the electromyograph (EMG), which measures muscular contraction and relaxation. Using biofeedback techniques, individuals can learn to control the firing of different motor units within a muscle and also the tension within whole muscles. An individual can learn the appropriate control of muscles, such as the frontalis in the forehead or the trapezius on the back, within a few hours. It is still uncertain whether such control can be maintained in the absence of the feedback.

EMG feedback has been used to retrain the muscles of the face following surgery, paralysis, various neck injuries and the condition known as spasmodic torticollis. It has also been applied in the treatment of tension headache, alleviation of anxiety symptoms and as an aid for poor readers. In most applications of muscle relaxation and neuromuscular re-education, however, it is still unknown how much control is maintained voluntarily once the biofeedback has ceased.

Research on biofeedback is now pointing the way to possible experimental approaches for testing it. Biofeedback is at least a highly provocative concept for understanding the interplay between the individual and the environment, and between the brain and its world. Investigations on self-control of the brain's electrical activity have centered on modification of the characteristics of the scalp electroencephalogram (EEG).

When electrodes are placed on the scalp, the resulting EEG consists of a number of different wave types. The first to be discovered was named the *alpha* wave. Although not the most frequently occurring one, it has sprung into prominence because of the biofeedback revolution. The alpha wave was first reported in 1924 by Hans Berger, a German psychiatrist who did further work on the alpha and beta waves throughout the early 1930s. Berger's descriptions of these waves were confirmed by Adrian and Matthews in 1934. Their paper was a catalyst for a rapid succession of other papers analyzing the alpha and beta waves and describing additional waves, including theta, delta and gamma waves.

Alpha waves have a frequency of 8-12 cycles per second. They are characteristic of states of rest and relief from attention and concentration. For many years it was thought that alpha waves appeared only when the eyes were closed, but that proved to be an oversimplification. Their presence in the EEG is associated with an alert but relaxed state of mind, and they generally appear in brief bursts rather than for a sustained period. Although their relationship to personality type is unclear, prominent alpha activity may be related to a dependent and submissive personality; minimal alpha activity may occur in hostile and aggressive individuals.

*Beta* waves, by contrast, have a frequency of 13-28 cycles per second and are characteristic of arousal. They appear during periods of intense concentration and mental agitation. Our fragmentary knowledge of beta waves is constantly being expanded. For instance, certain frequencies of beta waves occur normally during the early phases of sleep. As a whole, beta waves may be associated with processing visual information and with integrating information from diverse sources.

*Theta* waves, at 4-7 cycles per second, seem to be associated with emotionality, creative imagery, drowsiness, assimilation of new information and what is described as "computation on a deep level." They are not usually found in the waking EEG.

*Delta* waves at 0.5-3 cycles per second, are said to occur normally as a part of deep sleep. Abnormal ones may be associated with disease, degeneration and death.

In very experienced meditators the alpha waves are slower than normal (7-8 cycles per second as against 8-12) during meditation. As meditation proceeds it has been reported that alpha waves are replaced by fast-wave activity (40-45 cycles per second), which is followed by alpha and theta waves at a later stage.

Much attention has been focused on alpha biofeedback

because of its similarities to the brain-state of meditators. Yet the clinical relevance of EEG feedback should not be overlooked. In general, it is claimed to help those requiring mental relaxation, such as some people unable to sleep. More specifically, alpha training may help obsessive-compulsive neurotics, people with concentration and attention difficulties, and some cases of chronic pain. Overall, since EEG feedback is in its infancy, the possibility remains that the important therapeutic factor is not so much the alpha rhythm as general relaxation of the body. That development might have far-reaching implications for therapy and for the allure of meditation.

Biofeedback thus has a role to play in medical therapy. Although unorthodox in some regards, it is on the fringe of conventional medicine and may quite easily assume the trappings of orthodoxy. Before rushing in that direction, however, one should remember that it is a very new area of research, with most studies being little more than pilot investigations. Some studies have been inadequate and insufficiently controlled. We would be jumping to conclusions to hail biofeedback as the answer to all psychosomatic problems. Perhaps it will contribute to a new role of the patient in self-healing. It may extend the personal capacities of individuals in our technological culture. It might even mark the beginning of a new inward rather than outward direction for modern technology. But biofeedback is not without its dangers in making people even more dependent on impersonal technology. Further, the biofeedback boom is wide open for commercial exploitation by charlatans and unscrupulous businessmen.

Biofeedback edges us toward the frontiers of a new state of consciousness. If it achieves its results on muscle tension, heart rate or alpha rhythm by inducing an altered state of consciousness, it may have philosophical and religious as well as physiological implications. Barbara Brown, for instance, emphasizes the ability of biofeedback to uncover superior mind abilities and to expand awareness. The clinical dimensions are more prosaic and far more sober. Increased control of one's own body through one's own resources is surely a welcome development in an impersonal technological culture. But is an entirely new conceptual reality equally welcome?

## Transcendental Meditation (TM)

In a world of high technology and restless dissatisfaction, the Science of Creative Intelligence (SCI) and its practical technique, transcendental meditation (TM), are being put forward as *the* effective method of unfolding full human potential. They are said to combine Western scientific methods of objective investigation with the ancient wisdom of subjective development proclaimed in the Vedas. Advocates of TM claim that it frees people from the restrictions of stress, thereby allowing individuals to enjoy life more fully. Advocates point to studies showing increased learning ability, marked decrease in drug, alcohol and tobacco usage, increase of creativity and personal stability, quicker reaction time and reduced anxiety, neuroticism and crime. It is frequently even claimed that, in cities where more than one per cent of the population is practicing TM, the quality of life as a whole is improved—the so-called Maharishi effect.

The apparently limitless benefits of TM, at least according to TM literature, are said to stem from an experience of "pure" or "transcendental" consciousness, in which subjects feel fully awake and alert but are completely at rest. That is the crux of TM's credentials, which inevitably brings us to the interaction between TM and the brain.

R. Keith Wallace, professor of physiology and president of Maharishi International University (M.I.U.) at Fairfield, Iowa, states that the most ancient system for the development of consciousness has been reestablished in its purest and most effective form by Maharishi Mahesh Yogi, as the Science of Creative Intelligence. Wallace claims the system is being expressed in a way that makes it fully accessible to modern scientific techniques of investigation. TM is said to be a way for individuals to increase the functional integrity and orderliness of body and mind, and to extend the quality of being alive to its ultimate value. That, according to Wallace, is the equivalent of "enlightenment."

The history of TM is brief. TM originated in 1958 and acquired its impetus in 1965 with the formation of the Students' International Meditation Society in the United States. Its founder, Maharishi Mahesh Yogi, inaugurated a "world plan" in 1972 with seven goals. Among them are development of the full potential of the individual; solution of the problems of crime, drug abuse and all behavior that brings unhappiness; fulfillment of the economic aspirations of individuals and society; and achievement of the spiritual goals of mankind in this generation.

TM is constantly put forward as a nonreligious technique, which has enabled it to gain rapid acceptance by educational and government bodies in many Western countries. Almost one million people in the United States alone have been taught TM since 1965. The world plan calls for establishment of 3,600 centers for teaching the Science of Creative Intelligence around the world, approximately one center for every million people. Each center, in turn, is to train one teacher for every thousand people.

Allied to TM's allegedly nonreligious stance is its aura of scientific authenticity. It claims to counteract the pernicious effects of illicit drugs and anxiety and to provide the way to a healthier, more fulfilled life. These claims led the U.S. government at one time to fund research grants for the study of TM. TM was also adopted as an extracurricular course by certain American schools and as a recommended course for the employees of various corporations.

The two elements of TM—its nonreligious and scientific aspects—require separate discussion, although there is overlap between them. Let us first look at its scientific credentials.

The classic physiological studies of the effects of TM on bodily systems, carried out in the late 1960s by Wallace and Herbert Benson, were published in 1971 and '72. Wallace, now at M.I.U., has continued with experimental studies of TM. Wallace and Benson found, in subjects under-

*Figure 7.2 Indices commonly used to demonstrate some of the physiological consequences of TM, the measurements comparing levels before, during and after a meditation session. Intensity refers to the level of alpha waves in an EEG. Adapted from "The Physiology of Meditation." Copyright © 1972 by Scientific American, Inc. All rights reserved.*

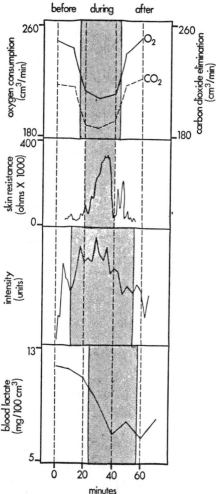

going TM, a reduction in oxygen consumption and carbon dioxide elimination, both trends reflecting a lower rate of respiration (Fig. 7.2). Blood pressure is also reduced, and a major fall in blood lactate concentration indicates decreased muscle metabolism. Skin resistance increases markedly, and cardiac output decreases by as much as 25 per cent. EEG recordings from the brain show an abundance of alpha waves, indicating a relaxed and comfortable state (Fig. 7.2).

The reason for the huge fall in lactate levels appears to be a correspondingly increased blood flow to the forearm muscles during meditation. The vessels obviously dilate, a result of activity of the autonomic nervous system. In view of the high blood lactate levels in patients with anxiety neurosis and hypertension, Wallace and Benson conclude that "the low level of lactate found in subjects during and after transcendental meditation may be responsible in part for the meditators' thoroughly relaxed state."

The large increase in galvanic skin resistance (GSR) is also said to indicate a high level of relaxation and calm (Fig. 7.2). Further studies on the GSR have indicated that meditators adjust to repeated stress more quickly than nonmeditators. That is again taken to signify the calmness of meditators.

From data such as these it has been concluded that TM can be distinguished from sleeping and dreaming on the one hand, and from hypnosis, biofeedback and autosuggestion on the other. The physiological and biochemical changes occurring during TM are described as relieving the strains and stresses accumulated on the nervous system more efficiently than either dreaming or sleeping. Wallace and Benson conclude that the state produced by TM is a *wakeful, hypometabolic one* in which quiescence rather than hyperactivation predominates.

Maharishi Mahesh Yogi has described that state as restful alertness which, in his view, represents the body's most healthy state and constitutes the basis of all energy and action. The condition has also been referred to as a fourth major state of consciousness, termed transcendental or pure consciousness. It is described as a state of silent awareness, devoid of any thought processes. That state has also been defined as the direct personal experience of the level of reality responsible for the structure of matter, energy and the laws governing physical events. The deep rest of TM allows the attention to fall on increasingly more refined, quieter levels of mental activity, until a point is allegedly

*Figure 7.3* *Schematic illustration of the belief that TM leads to a state of pure consciousness. The deep rest of TM is claimed to turn the mind away from action toward the source of thought, "being" itself. This model is offered in the teachings of Maharishi Mahesh Yogi and the TM movement. Adapted from Jack Forem,* Transcendental Meditation: Maharishi Mahesh Yogi and the Science of Creative Intelligence, © *1974. Used by permission of the author.*

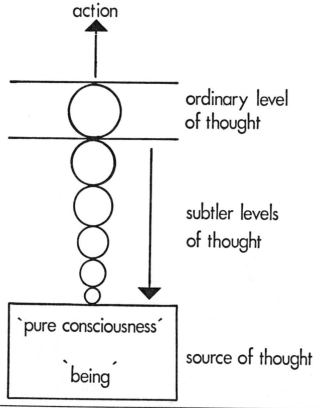

action

ordinary level
of thought

subtler levels
of thought

`pure consciousness`

`being`

source of thought

reached in which even the faintest thought is transcended and the subject remains wide awake and yet not attending to anything (Fig. 7.3).

When TM is described in such terms, one wonders if it is still appropriate to talk about it from a scientific viewpoint. There is no doubt that TM has extremely interesting and perhaps highly unusual physiological consequences; it is another matter to argue that it ushers in a unique state of consciousness. Repeatedly in the writings of TM exponents one comes across a jump from orthodox physiological approaches and conventional scientific language to non-scientific concepts. For instance, the absence of random GSR fluctuations and the appearance of EEG synchrony (characteristics of sleep or rest) are said to reinforce the view that low metabolic activity generates an increase of orderliness in central nervous system function. Yet it is far from clear what "orderliness" in the central nervous system means. "Growth in consciousness" is an equally ambiguous phrase.

On the other hand, such terminology has much in common with the "cosmic consciousness" of the new-consciousness movement. In cosmic consciousness, explanations are essentially metaphysical rather than scientific, since the self and the cosmos supposedly become of a piece, and at times are even united. Fulfillment stems from oneness with the universe, which in turn derives from a fundamental re-ordering of an individual's view of reality. Encompassed by that reordering is an emphasis on the mind as the all-controlling reality at the heart of the physical universe, plus a belief that whatever the self perceives and believes actually exists. When TM is taken to its limits, as in the Sidhi program discussed below, it becomes a vehicle for alteration of states of consciousness. In the realm of the transcendent, a person may no longer be in control of his or her own mind.

Certain claims of TM soon take it out of the realm of the scientific. Nevertheless, it is worth referring to a number of other scientific studies. A few studies have been aimed at tracing biochemical and hormonal changes in groups of subjects before learning the TM technique and after months of practice at the technique, and in regular participants in the TM program. Parameters measured have included plasma cortisol, lactate, phenylalanine, prolactin, epinephrine and norepinephrine levels. Some evidence from these studies suggests that the TM technique can be distinguished from other hypometabolic states, although other evidence is equivocal. Another avenue of approach has been to measure levels of cortisol and various transmitter metabolites excreted in the urine of subjects. Although differences have been noted between meditators and nonmeditators, the significance of the differences is a matter for debate.

The conflicting nature of the results just mentioned is rather typical of most of the evidence on TM. Studies not in agreement with TM-favorable reports are rarely mentioned in TM literature; adequate controls have not always been incorporated into investigations. No doubt relaxation plays a large part in many of the supposedly beneficial effects of TM, as do the expectations of the meditators. Another possibility, about which little is heard, is that TM—if practiced to excess—may do harm, especially in people with a tendency toward mental illness. For instance, an extremely anxious person may find that in the deep calm of meditation problems rather than solutions are encountered.

The influence of TM on the brain has been analyzed almost entirely by EEG changes. Certain aspects of these changes have already been mentioned, such as an increase in alpha activity in meditators. Beta and high-amplitude theta spindles have also been observed, the theta activity being regular and unlike that found in the onset of sleep. Coefficients of wakefulness (alpha:delta) and of activation (beta:alpha) have been used to distinguish TM, with its decreased activation and increased wakefulness, from both drowsiness and sleep. With experience at TM, it is claimed that transcendental consciousness persists during the waking state, a process referred to by Maharishi as the growth of cosmic consciousness. That process, allegedly the basis of the beneficial social and health features of TM, is said to be brought about by "the formation of facilitated neural pathways which ultimately enable the state of pure consciousness to persist in the presence of waking activity in the state of cosmic consciousness." With such a claim we are back once more at TM's metaphysical base.

The postulated consequences of that circumstance for individual health are almost unlimited. Beside the alleged benefits already referred to, evidence is claimed to show improvements in academic performance, organization of memory, intelligence growth rate, job performance and satisfaction, and self-actualization. Improvement is also claimed in such medical conditions as migraine, diabetes, low back pain, phobic disorders, stuttering and allergic disorders. It is even claimed that TM can reverse the normal aging process by introducing into the body the principles of adaptability, stability, integration, purification and growth. Such "definitive properties of pure consciousness" allow above-average performance in many body systems.

In the claims of TM we see the ease with which orthodox scientific concepts have been transmuted into an idealistic framework for a highly unorthodox form of holistic medicine. We should be concerned not so much with the dichotomy between orthodoxy and unorthodoxy as with the manner in which terminology and concepts have been radically transformed. What is put forward as a simple, nondemanding technique is in fact a revolutionary philosophical about-face. The "perfect health" and "higher state of consciousness" of TM are harbingers of a world view that has much in common with certain forms of Hindu mysticism, despite the repeated claim of TM apologists that it is a nonreligious technique.

The TM-Sidhi program, which has been available since early 1977, is said to open the way to the direct experience of higher states of consciousness. That depends on the ability to maintain transcendental consciousness simultaneously with waking activity. Essential for that development is a state of "unity consciousness," an extension of cosmic consciousness and a state in which sensory perception is said to become increasingly acute. It is argued that this state conveys an ability to alter the objective world by intention so that objects outside one's own body can be influenced as readily as can the systems of one's own body. Capabilities stemming from that ability, collectively known as *Sidhis,* include levitation, perceiving the location of objects hidden from view and rendering oneself invisible. Sidhis are taken as evidence of more complete integration of mind and body. They illustrate the new-consciousness viewpoint that the self is in charge of everything; whatever it wishes to believe, *is.* As any distinction between appearance and reality vanishes, a person is free to believe anything he or she likes because no view of reality is more real than any other. At that point we see TM expressing the essence of cosmic consciousness.

Whatever the validity of the Sidhi phenomena and whatever their effects on the subjects themselves, they take us into the realms of mystical experience. Perhaps the major difference between TM and many other forms of mysticism is that TM claims scientific validation of its procedures. It attempts to provide scientific justification for the directions in which it is moving. It purports to have demonstrated that the TM program has transformed the study of consciousness into a major scientific field and has pointed medical research in a new direction. It presents itself, therefore, as an alternative to scientific medicine as we know it, with its own form of wholeness and well-being as the basis of individual and societal health.

Convincing and enticing as some of these claims may sound, the presuppositions on which they are built cannot be ignored. Like mood-affecting drugs, TM aims to modify the perception of the individual rather than the social situation. Alleviation of stress, therefore, is effected without any reference at all to the cause of the stress, and results from just forty minutes of meditation a day. TM seeks to change the state of consciousness rather than the condition of the external world. If enough people's consciousnesses are changed the quality of life of their society will be changed. A Westerner finds it difficult to accept the rationale of that view until it is seen as the logical outworking of the Hindu notion that we project the material universe into existence by our collective consciousness of it.

TM represents a combination of Eastern and Western concepts which can be readily assimilated into a middle-class, capitalist society. TM produces individuals who accept everything in society as a *given*. Then TM adjusts the perceptions and reactions of these individuals, thereby enabling them to accept more readily their lot within society. TM bestows apparent peace and contentment without disrupting a person's participation in, or commitment to, the systems of society. It allows "transcendence" without alienation.

TM lacks the radicalness of a truly human response in which the person *and* the situation are changed—since the situation may be at fault rather than the person. Although TM may dispense with psychotropic drugs, its action has many similarities to that of such drugs. Instead of chemical modification of the brain, TM—at least in its more "advanced" forms—is modifying the brain and its perception of reality by psychological and semireligious means.

The base of TM is indisputably religious. Its essential principle is that the relative and the absolute are brought together into a cosmic union. Integration of life's inner and outer phases is, however, an example of *monism,* the doctrine of the unity of all being.

The initiation ceremony for novice meditators, when they offer flowers, fruit and a handkerchief to Guru Dev and receive their *mantra,* contains an invocation in Sanskrit. In part, that hymn reads: "To Lord Narayana, to lotus-born Brahma, the Creator, to Vashista ... I bow down. At whose door the whole galaxy of gods pray for perfection day and night. Adorned with immeasurable glory, preceptor of the whole world, having bowed down to him we gain fulfillment."

That procedure is like a traditional Hindu worship ceremony, the particular tradition being that of a Hindu master named Shankara. The principal focus of worship is a successor of Shankara, the late Brahmananda Saraswati or Gurù Dev. The link to the Maharishi Mahesh Yogi is direct: Guru Dev was his master.

In the initiation, under the form of Guru Dev (whose picture is on the altar), the Hindu Trimurti of Brahma, Vishnu and Shiva are being worshiped as manifestations of the formless absolute, Brahman. Thus we have an almost classic expression of a foundational principle of Eastern pantheistic monism, that Atman is Brahman—the soul of man is the Soul of the cosmos. Both Atman and Brahman are impersonal, implying that humanity in its truest, fullest being is impersonal. For human beings to realize their being they must learn to enter the undifferentiated, impersonal cosmic One.

TM's stress on pure consciousness is consistent with its monistic base. The ordinary states of consciousness—waking, dreaming and deep sleep—must be transcended in order to attain union with the unity of the cosmos. Pure consciousness, therefore, is pure being, rather than any state of consciousness with which physiologists are familiar. Each self is potentially the universe; cosmic consciousness implies the unity of all reality. That unity must extend beyond moral distinctions as well as metaphysical ones.

Perhaps that is the reason why TM makes no moral demands on meditators except for the initiation ban on alcohol and drugs. TM is thus at odds with many Eastern religions, which demand rigorous discipline and practice from their adherents. TM is typical of the new-consciousness movement in that regard.

Our discussion has brought us beyond the bounds of science and the brain. Nevertheless, we have gone no further than the territories staked out by TM. It is true that for the vast majority of those who indulge in TM, many of whom persevere for only a few months, TM is nothing more than a relaxation technique. Its essence and rationale, however, are far more profound, constituting a monistic answer to the depersonalization of modern life which is the legacy of secularistic materialism. That answer conflicts head-on with Christianity in its views of God, of human nature, and of redemption. The fundamental distinction between Creator and creature, so essential to the biblical revelation of God, disappears in TM's postulates of the unity of all being. Redemption, instead of arising from God's initiative in Christ's Incarnation, is found in an individual's efforts to attain unity with the essence of being. The grace of God is replaced by people's self-sufficiency to experience their own divinity. The role of science has also been transmuted; instead of an implement to help human beings exert responsible dominion over the created order, it is used to demonstrate that they can transcend their nature by acquiring "pure consciousness."

## Individual Consciousnesses

Earlier in this chapter we saw that, to a person such as Charles Tart, our culture must transcend its mechanistic approach before we can begin to realize the scope of human potential. That means that science as we know it must change. Its focus must shift from the external world to internal experience, to the realm of altered perception and discrete altered states of consciousness. The end result of such radical transformation might be, according to Tart, different sciences with different perspectives on reality—perhaps not more or less true than ordinary-state science, but complementary to it.

Do Tart's ideas make sense? One attempt to give them validity has been made by John Lilly, a neurophysiologist recognized for his work with dolphins. During the 1950s, Lilly started experimenting with LSD and sensory deprivation. In the sensory deprivation experiments, Lilly subjected himself to periods of isolation, lying buoyant in fluid in a darkened, closed tank. With all external stimuli reduced as much as possible, the mind begins to generate its own inputs and the subject has "out-of-the-body experiences." Using his LSD-isolation tank model, Lilly began explorations into the way the mind operates in various states of consciousness. After years of such experiments, combined with other meditative exercises, Lilly has become a cartographer of altered states of consciousness. One of his best-known books, *The Center of the Cyclone*, subtitled *An Autobiography of Inner Space*, is described by Lilly as "an open-ended, open-minded metatheory of the supraconscious, expanded-awareness states."

Lilly's explorations into mind-brain relations are based on the belief that nonordinary states of consciousness exist and that it is possible to get into them. The premise is that in the realm of the mind, what one believes to be true becomes true within certain limits, the limits to be found experientially and experimentally. In turn, these limits are further beliefs to be transcended; in the mind, there *are* no limits. Believing that, Lilly is a typical new-consciousness exponent. Elevating the self and the mind, he expects unlimited vistas to open up to him so he can wander through one space after another and one universe after another.

To follow Lilly a little way will help us appreciate the compelling attraction and transforming power of these spaces for someone with his basic postulates. In his initial "trips," Lilly saw himself as a single point of consciousness, being taught by two "guardians" about the "reality" of the inner spaces of the mind. He describes these two guides as two aspects of his own functioning at the supraself level; not knowing their precise identity, he recognizes them as in some sense setting goals for him in his supraself journeys. With further experience he came to accept that "all and everything that one can imagine exists"; that acceptance enabled him to indulge freely in his new spaces, having overcome any fear of leaving his body behind.

As he learned to enter the spaces where his guardians existed, he became increasingly dependent on their advice.

They advised him to return to his body and to perfect means of communicating with those spaces, for example. While doing further experiments he was aware of his guides' presence. At one point he felt they were showing him the whole universe and indicating humanity's place in it. The more he experienced the LSD-isolation-induced mental states, the more convinced he became of their reality. His own succinct description is "I knew that this was the truth." In later years he experimented with hypnotic trances and meditative exercises, but the essence of his explorations is summed up in his initial trips.

Several other features of Lilly's trips are significant. His own subjective feelings during or immediately after these experiences were responses of awe, reverence and a sense of smallness. Following one experience he wrote: "Everything was happening on such a vast scale that I was merely an observer of microscopic size, and yet I was more than this. I was part of some vast network of similar beings all connected . . . I was given an individuality for temporary purposes only. I would be reabsorbed into the network when the time came." After some trips he regretted having to return to his body and ordinary consciousness.

Lilly's visits to inner space, however, were not all light and warmth. He also experienced what he described as alien, demonic forms pouring into a "hole" in his head. It was as if he were at an interface between two universes, one characterized by golden light and love and warmth, the other by a dark, threatening cloud of evil. The blackness and pain of that latter universe filled him with terror, his answer to which was to find the space where his two guides resided. Significantly, perhaps, one of the black occasions coincided with a migraine attack during the period of his altered state of consciousness.

Coming from a Roman Catholic background, Lilly had dispensed with any religious beliefs and had become instead a mechanistic, atheistic scientist. His pattern of complacent nonbelief was shattered, however, by his altered states of consciousness. To him, his lack of belief became a limiting belief. After one particularly punishing experience, he was deeply grieved and profoundly moved; he began to consider that there must be a guiding intelligence in the universe, and that God existed in him. His experiences with the guides were, for him, a shared, organized aspect of the universe; he came to feel that the negative aspects of his science had kept him away from humanity. Not long after that, in 1969, he resigned from his scientific position and started a new life.

Although Lilly has touched on various meditative programs, he remains a "scientific explorer," shunning dogmatism and worship, but seeking instead insight into universal nature and our own inner natures. Deeply committed to the "highest" states of consciousness, Lilly concludes *The Center of the Cyclone* with these words: "The miracle is that the universe created a part of itself to study the rest of it, that this part, in studying itself, finds the rest of the universe in its own natural inner realities."

Lilly clearly illustrates the transformation that must take place if dependence on ordinary consciousness is replaced by other forms of consciousness. In particular he gives us insight into what an "altered-state-of-consciousness" type of science might mean. It is a "science" in which the experimenter becomes the center of the experiment, in which the subjective displaces almost completely any hint of the objective. Lilly refrains from worship, insisting that his task is to map the geography of inner space and other universes. Yet even for him, that is an intensely *personal* and lonely journey. One suspects that the terrain being covered is the terrain of John Lilly's mind, rather than the terrain of the human mind. One of the basic tenets of the new consciousness was noted by James Sire in *The Universe Next Door*, namely, that the prime reality in that movement is the *self*. Sire describes the movement's outlook: "The external universe exists not to be manipulated from the outside by a transcendent God but to be manipulated from the inside by the self."

Science, for Lilly, has become a natural history of his own mind while in an altered state of consciousness. There can be no doubt that it is vastly different from conventional science. How can it warrant the name *science* at all? It has become a description of mystical visions. Any such description can be called "The science of belief" as Lilly calls them in his book *Simulations of God*. Lilly's form of science is based on the belief that one view of reality is as good as another, and one symbol system is as valid as any other.

Clearly, however, Lilly's science is a science of an internal and normally invisible universe. Its validity is not subject to the tests applicable to the external, visible universe. Even if one accepted its validity, Lilly's "science" would be irrelevant for the world of ordinary consciousness, in which even Lilly has to spend much of his waking time. The multitude of sciences required to describe the multitude of "realities" stemming from altered states of consciousness cannot, therefore, invalidate the rationale of science developed for "ordinary-state-of-consciousness" activities. That brings us back to the personal nature of Lilly's science and to its inability to serve the needs of humanity at large.

A view of the nature of *reality* as *relative* lies at the heart of Lilly's science. He has no assurance that external reality is more real than internal reality. Indeed, when in one of the altered mental states, he feels their reality so intensely that he questions the existence of his body and of his place in the material universe. That uncertainty stems from uncertainty about the mind-brain relationship. Lilly gives predominance to the mind, with its freedom to explore universes of its own making. The brain has become a valve through which the mind speaks.

By isolating the mind from the brain in that manner, Lilly negates the brain's significance. It was consistent for him, therefore, to give up his work as a neuroscientist. When the mind is exalted, the brain becomes little more than an object of curiosity, a material phenomenon of limited interest. Lilly's denigration of the material realm is a heresy as ancient as Gnosticism. The terminology has changed, but the essence is the same. For Lilly, the brain is limiting, whereas the mind is open to adventures of endless possibilities. Our ordinary state of consciousness seems mundane and narrow in contrast to altered states of consciousness with their un-dreamed-of worlds and limitless horizons. The brain, then the body, then all aspects of the material creation become unimportant.

To demean the creation is to demean the work of God as Creator and the Incarnation of Christ in coming to redeem the creation. In elevating the human mind, Lilly gives to creatures a creatorial role: the creation of a world of their own imagining. A Christian can see that as a vain attempt to escape the bondage of a sinful world, with its limitations, responsibilities and challenge. The mind is not a means of escaping the consequences of a bodily existence, but the expression of what human beings can think, create and be as creatures created in the image of God. To manipulate the mind as if it were a plaything is to deny the rational side of what it means to be human.

A final aspect of Lilly's version of the new consciousness to consider is his use of the concept of God. One finds no hint that he accepts the existence of a transcendent God. Rather, his version of God appears to depend on the state of his own consciousness. Essentially, however, he sees himself as a programmer of the cosmic computer, a god under God, re-sponsible for running the universe. He creates energy, mat-ter and life at the interface between the void and all known creation. He is the *creation process* itself: "one of the boys in the engine room pumping creation from the void into the known universe."

Hence, Lilly *is* God; he is in control of his own universe, creating it and tending it. For us, his universe is nothing more than a figment of one person's imagination. For him, it is as real as any other universe, and he is God. That is the ultimate impasse of the new consciousness: reality and God become nothing more than internal constructs. There is no

God except me, because there is no reality except me and no universe except me. All that remains for Lilly and those like him are experiences; nothing else exists because they have made everything relative. The end result can only be nihilism, in which all traditional notions of freedom, dignity and ethical absolutes have been abandoned.

## The Analytical and the Intuitive

The new consciousness has as its basis a multiplicity of realities. Whether there are two or innumerable realities, the principle is the same: the "other" forms of realities are the ones on which practical and religious emphasis is placed.

The choice between two forms of reality is made clear by Robert Ornstein in his analysis of meditation. The choice, in his words, is between two modes of consciousness, the analytical and the intuitive; others use different descriptions for what are probably the same two consciousness forms. On occasions the choice is between intellectual and personal knowledge, or between active and quiescent modes. Simplistically, we may think of it as left-hemisphere and right-hemisphere functioning, although as we saw in chapter 2, the situation is not that straightforward.

According to Ornstein, *meditation* is a set of techniques aimed at inhibiting the usual mode of consciousness and cultivating a second mode. That is accomplished by dismantling the automaticity and selectivity of ordinary awareness, which then leads to a reduction of the normal selectivity of input. The nonordinary mode of consciousness, therefore, lacks the normal construction of ordinary consciousness, a shift having taken place from an analytical, piecemeal approach to knowledge to a more receptive, holistic mode. It is further argued by Ornstein that the mystic experience lies outside the province of language and rationality, and is complementary to the ordered sequence of normal thought. Not only that, it adds comprehension to the ordinary mode.

The reasons why people seek mystical experiences include a desire to encompass aspects of experience outside the analytical. At a deeper level, some long to enter into the unity and expanse of the universe, the longing eloquently expressed by John Lilly. The deautomatization implicit in meditative techniques is claimed to open a person to factors he or she has previously ignored. That is the basis of meditation's positive virtues.

That argument requires serious consideration. Both analysis and intuition are essential for human existence in all its fullness; a choice should not have to be made between them. Both ways of thinking are required to solve the problems of individuals and society. An adequate appreciation of the world requires both modes. A balanced, healthy existence for individuals is dependent on both. Normal family and social life are possible only when both modes are utilized.

Certain aspects of Western civilization, such as its materialism and secularism, may well be consequences of an almost exclusive regard for analytical abilities. The secularism characterizing much Western science until the 1950s viewed scientific analysis as the sole legitimate approach to reality. The tide is now turning strongly against such reductionism, with due regard being paid to ascientific, nonanalytical approaches to the world. The time has perhaps come for a thorough study of intuition-based systems of thought. The place to start may well be with the organization of our brains.

What is the place of religious approaches to the world? It is fascinating to speculate on the demands that Christian thinking makes on brain function. After all, Christians—motivated by biblical precepts—played a major part in the rise of modern science, yet Christianity also depends on a nonanalytical acceptance of the world as a God-breathed fact. The blend of the analytical and the intuitive should come to fruition in the lives of individual Christians and in the Christian community as a whole.

Any demands for an outlook based solely on impersonal analysis are hollow. Such an approach fails to provide a world of meaning, and lacks understanding of the nature of human beings as multifaceted creatures. The many sides to our personalities are a strength rather than a weakness. We must be able to show firmness and strength, love and compassion; we must be capable of thinking critically and perceptively, while also indulging in humor and inconsequential wit. Wholeness of experience and response stems from a oneness within our brains; it is a left-hemisphere *and* right-hemisphere response combined. The Christian response demands wholeness of personality and an acceptance of our limitations as well as possibilities.

Many forms of meditation, however, go far beyond a view of the complementarity of the two modes of consciousness. The new-consciousness movement seeks a radical reappraisal of the religious basis of Western culture and of its dependence on a rational, ordered approach to reality. Such a reappraisal would highlight nonrationality and lack of order. Desire for unity and oneness would overshadow distinctions between the Creator and his creatures. Taken to those limits, the new consciousness shows clearly an espousal of pantheistic, mystical overtones rather than Judeo-Christian thought. The choice is ultimately religious, not merely the narrow choice of analysis versus intuition. All new-consciousness trends should be viewed in that light, whatever their claims.

The new-consciousness movement turns the spotlight on both strengths and weaknesses within Western culture. In rejecting weaknesses, such as excessive regard for the analytical, the movement is in grave danger of rejecting the strengths, such as concern for a systematic approach to a world regarded as capable of rational explanation. At times Western culture has replaced the rational with "rationalism," producing a morass of antisupernaturalism and deification of "autonomous man." It is right to reject such rationalism, but to replace it with intuitive "irrationalism" will produce a system in which the irrational itself is deified.

The new-consciousness movement also represents a backlash against technology and impersonalism. Robert Ornstein, in his assessment of biofeedback, says:

> The research so far in biofeedback marks the merest beginnings of a new attempt to turn the direction of modern technology itself inward, away from the control and manipulation of the external environment. Just as technology has often limited man's personal capacities, so it can also extend them. Technology itself is neutral, and can be employed to make man less or more human. In the feedback paradigm technology has been refocused towards an extension of our own personal capacities, rather than a diminution of them.

Christians should welcome a concern for human beings as *persons* and a concern for a technology that serves human beings rather than manipulates them. Such Christian concerns have been voiced by Professor Jacques Ellul in *The Technological Society.* For Ellul, "technique" is a principle made out of a process, a mentality made out of a machine, the translation into action of the human wish to master things by reason alone. As a consequence, artificiality is increased. The natural environment is giving way to a technological one, while technology itself is on the way to assuming autonomy. Technique's autonomy constitutes the basis of Ellul's opposition to it. Not only is autonomous technology outside human control, but it subverts social values, relegates the individual to a position of subservience and elevates technical expertise to the position of dominant control in human affairs.

Against that background a desire to turn technology inward is understandable. Nevertheless, both the technological and mystical revolutions require analysis. The guiding principle of such analysis from a Christian standpoint should be that any revolution must serve human beings rather than injure them. It is imperative that the "brain revolution" raise our respect for humanity and not diminish it. We need wholeness, not fragmentation; fulfillment, not shallowness. In a quest for expanded consciousness, we need a model of what expanded consciousness might imply.

For the Christian, a model is at hand: the example of Jesus. In him we have the perfect blend of humanity and divinity, and hence the perfect amalgam of human and transcendental consciousness. Christ was able to live human life to the full, living out the best in human life within the broader context of the divine perspective. He was no less than God and man in one person.

Yet Jesus Christ is not simply a model, because a model by itself may daunt. Jesus Christ is actually *the way* into what could be called a "new consciousness," by virtue of his divine-human status. He demonstrates to us our limited consciousness, then provides us with a means of expanding it through our knowledge of God and through a new life in himself. That is what Christians refer to as the new birth; it is indeed an expansion of consciousness—and a renewal of life itself.

# 8

## The Human Brain and the Human Person

OUR TASK IN THIS FINAL CHAPTER is to examine the relationship between a person's brain and what makes that person the sort of being she or he is. If a person is no more than a brain, there is no place for "mind" or perhaps even for personhood. Alternatively, to strive to accommodate mind within a contemporary neurobiological view of the brain is no easy task—as we shall see.

### The Demise of the Mind

The extreme complexity of the human brain daunts many people and sometimes proves too much even for neuroscientists. Nevertheless, piece by piece, the brain is being described in rudimentary, material terms. True, we have a very long way to go before we can realistically say that we *understand* the brain scientifically. Yet research fervor in the neurosciences continues, and without doubt the reductionism of that approach is paying dividends.

The debit side of that reductionism is the demise of the person. Increasingly, human behavior can be accounted for without recourse to any explanation drawing on the conscious decisions of persons. As a result of that trend, it has become increasingly difficult to view persons as *responsible* agents. Actions and beliefs appear to be explainable by neurobiological concepts. When that procedure is taken to logical extremes, no room is left for personhood, freedom or responsibility; everything is related directly to a person's brain. The person becomes subordinated to the brain, understood in the limited, physical categories of scientific causality.

Of course, one cannot escape the centrality of the brain for an understanding of ourselves as persons. To deny this is to ignore many of the data encountered in the preceding chapters. Whatever we conceive ourselves to be is intimately related to the state of our brain—and can be modified by a variety of assaults on our brain. We are not "islands unto ourselves" for the simple reason that our brains are not islands unto themselves. Such a potentially mechanistic view of the brain often alarms people for two main reasons.

In the first place it highlights the *fragility* of our brains. In no sense is the brain immune to outside pressures, including inimical ones. To some people, any type of brain research poses a major threat to the brain's integrity and hence to us as persons. A brain so vulnerable to outside assault is open to manipulation by other persons. Some possibilities for manipulation have been touched on earlier.

A second cause for concern in the face of a potentially mechanistic view of the brain stems from the question mark it places beside many traditional views of *human responsibility*. When the brain is viewed in machinelike terms, it is a short step to the conclusion that a human being actually *is* a machine. If the brain comes to be regarded as a glorified computer, any person can be seen as a complex array of interacting gadgetry. If we are *nothing but* machines, and if our brains are as determined as clockwork toys, how can we any longer be regarded as free agents?

Obviously, a mechanistic description of human beings and the brain may herald the demise of the person—and of the mind. In principle, the mechanistic approach appears capable of explaining the whole of brain structure and function, and consequently of behavior, without any reference to the mind. A thoroughgoing mechanist might hold that mind as a discernible, separate entity does not exist, or that if it does exist it has to be viewed in radical ways. Perhaps at that point we must call the all-encompassing nature of mechanistic description into question.

The validity and content of the concept of mind will occupy our attention in the next three sections. First we shall consider certain consequences of the demise of the concept by referring to the views of two contemporary biologists.

For psychologist B. F. Skinner, man can be known only by analyzing him psychologically. That analysis alone provides the data for Skinner's view of man; nothing else is considered legitimate. As Skinner himself remarks, man is more like a dog than a god because he can be scientifically analyzed like a dog—whereas a god belongs to the realm of the metaphysical and fictional. Scientific analysis is allowable and good; metaphysics is neither, to Skinner.

Skinner exults in man's machinelike nature and in the abolition of what he terms "autonomous man." By that term he means the idea that human beings in some way stand in contrast to the impersonal cosmic machine, able to make real choices and to know that they are free. To Skinner there is no such freedom; he wants to dispense with the notion that man has a body with a person inside, because to him man *is* a body which *is* a person which *is* a complex repertoire of behavior. There is no such thing as "man in his humanity," therefore; there is only "man the machine."

For Skinner, a human being is a set of behavioral responses. What is more, he argues, since these responses are open to modification by the environment, man is controlled by the world around him. The environment which is manmade is as much in control of man, therefore, as is man of the environment.

One might conclude that human beings, in Skinner's eyes, are hopeless creatures trapped in a world of their own devices. Far from it; there are wonderful possibilities opening up to them. Application of technological expertise, rather than trapping human beings, opens up many possibilities for changing them. Using positive reinforcers and seeing the environment as all-important in laying down behavior patterns, Skinner envisages inducing people to behave well by rewarding them appropriately, control being exercised by society through the techniques of behaviorism.

In Skinner's utopian technocracy, conditioning and a technology of behavior are the only guiding principles. In that form of "the science of man" there is no room for mind or freedom; we are left with manipulation of the environment and subsequent behavioral acquiescence by conditioned people.

But if man is controlled by the environment and the environment is manmade, a question arises: Who directs the environment? The next question to arise is: What constitutes good and right actions in such a society? If human beings can be limitlessly manipulated, one needs some assurance that the ethics underlying the manipulation are "good."

So, what are good ethics, and how can the foisting of arbitrary ethical systems on a population be justified? In the limited space of this book, we can only comment that the rightness or wrongness of ethical systems presupposes the existence of man as a free and responsible being, a concept denounced by Skinner. Someone has to decide the *direction* in which society is to go; someone has to make *value* judgments; someone must be *free* to decide. But such freedom is found only in full human beings.

Even a society based on psychological conditioning, therefore, must resort to certain individuals utilizing a wide range of human capacities. Skinner's arguments lead us to the question of the structure of society and the extent to which an elite or the majority within a society is encouraged to function as responsible human beings. Skinner's society is based on the premise that its leaders will act *as though* they are free and responsible; otherwise there is no society.

Related to this consideration is the question of the justification of psychological conditioning. Skinner assumes that, if human beings are not free agents, manipulation based on conditioning is automatically acceptable. But that itself is a value judgment built into the behaviorist system.

It is useful for certain purposes to compare a human being to a machine. Between that useful methodological statement, however, and the assertion that "man is nothing but a machine" is a chasm of untold dimensions. The demise of human beings as responsible agents and the demise of the mind signify a move away from any serious concern with inner mental states to exclusive concern with behavior. Consequently, all values are based on their survival potential, so the individual becomes subservient to other individuals with more power in society. The demise of freedom leads inexorably to the demise of the dignity and equality of opportunity of individual human beings.

Skinner's utopian technocracy, with its linchpin of behavioral control, is a rather extreme example of the demise of the mind. A far more subtle, though less easily assimilated, example has been provided by J. Z. Young, a neuroscientist with far-reaching interests in applying his knowledge of the brain to understanding the human enterprise.

The essential theme of Young's book *Programs of the Brain* is that brains contain programs that regulate our lives. He proposes that the lives of human beings are governed by sets of programs written in their genes and brains. These programs, expressed in appropriate "languages" within the brain, are plans of action—each with its own desired goals. In such an argument, Young looks for a scheme with which to talk and think usefully about the brain. Young asserts that the programs provide the brain with a way of conducting life; they produce actions to keep the organism alive. They provide information stores not only for eating and sleeping but also for more complicated actions such as loving and hating, knowing and thinking, and even believing and worshiping. Programs of the brain, as plans for action, fit an individual for the ongoing task of coping with the demands of living.

Young then proceeds to work out the brain's role in such characteristically human responses as loving and caring, altruism and aggression, belief and faith, the experience of pleasure and pain. He analyzes every aspect of human existence solely in terms of the organization of the brain—without recourse to the mind.

Young is fully aware of dispensing with the concept of mind which, for him, is a term referring to "the system of operations of the programs of the brain of a person during conscious experience." Allowing that *mind* is a useful description of the brain's general mode of operation, he considers it at best a vague concept. Increased understanding of brain organization should lead to its replacement by other concepts depicting the modes of action of brain processes. With Young we have a major shift in emphasis away from the immaterial mind to the material brain. The shift seems dramatic because of Young's rigorous use of brain processes to grasp the *mysterium tremendum* of human existence.

For instance, Young uses the term *god,* but for him it has none of the supernatural, majestic, creatorial characteristics of the Hebraic-Christian view of God. Rather, it is a linguistic tool, simply a brain program necessary for understanding our beginnings. The program tells us little about the character of God because such information is not implicit within our brains. From Young's perspective, the starting point of all investigations about ourselves and our world is the codes, signs and languages used by our brains. He thus assumes a closed universe—one that is not open to the revelation of God. Yet the brain's programs are simply reflections of our heredity, early environment, culture and presuppositions as individuals; even our brains must be subject to the limitations imposed on us as finite beings.

For Young, religious belief, like art or music, is important because it has proved valuable for human survival. That means that religion assumes purely naturalistic overtones. Man's brain, instead of God's purpose, is the fulcrum of the universe.

The naturalistic basis of Young's position emerges repeatedly in *Programs of the Brain*. The existence of pleasure centers in the brain prompts him to propose that human aims and values can no longer be regarded as transcendental processes. They spring, he contends, from the effort to meet needs, since the programs we have inherited tell us to continue to promote life. Beliefs about human values are best studied, Young argues, by considering their origins, since values are the product of people and the reward centers of their brains. His view leaves in abeyance the issue of why reward centers developed in the first place and provides no clue to the criteria by which these centers operate.

Young has no desire to separate the question of how people think from what they think about. Nevertheless, his reliance on brain mechanisms as *the* rationale for understanding human existence makes that relationship tenuous. Reductionism is always close at hand, however valiantly Young may try to ward it off.

Having rejected a Christian position, Young is left with the unity of the whole brain program as his raison d'etre. He finds himself unable to reject either the order and purpose to life that seem evident from scientific investigations or the fact that many fundamental truths of life—pleasure and pain, beauty and worth—are not logically determined. Study of the brain suggests that all modes of truth are necessary to understand the brain as well as life itself.

That realization leads him to an acceptance of one's own life as fundamental, since life itself is the most enduring organized reality we know on earth. Hence, respect for life emerges as the central criterion by which every person's life is to be judged. For Young, realization that one exists, and *is,* lies at the heart of religious experience and forms the essence of worship. *To be,* and to be alive, are profoundly moving facets of the wonder of human existence.

Thus, in the context of the demise of the mind, we find a writer coming surprisingly close to a Christian position. Young is able to do that, perhaps, because of his view that the human brain functions as a unity. It follows that man, as a person, is a unity manifesting a wholeness one dare not ignore. Although Young is not prepared to allow a supernatural aspect to human existence, he grapples with the biological, personal, aesthetic, moral and belief facets of human life. In doing so he maintains most of the essential elements making up the *humanum.* It could be argued that he has maintained even the mind, albeit within a mechanistic framework.

Young's position, however, differs in fundamental ways from a Christian one. His view of belief and worship appears to ignore the evil and aggression in the human situation. Perhaps, when confronted by the need to find some ultimate meaning in human life, his optimism forces him to ignore evil. Christians rejoice at the wonder of life, but we also mourn at the evil in our midst. That is a tension with which we must live; to do otherwise is to reject a fundamental tenet of the world we experience. Christians can live with and understand such tension because the Christian world view incorporates a perfect creation, a Fall and a redemption. Young comes close to God the Creator, but misses altogether God the Redeemer. Yet it is in these two facets of God that we begin to appreciate what wholeness means. And as we look at the outworking of God's power through the Holy Spirit, we see more fully that the unity of the Godhead is fundamental to the wholeness of human life.

In summary, one can argue that Young's final position fails to do justice to his mechanistic premises. There are indications that he has made his own leap of faith in order to maintain the integrity of the human person. To accomplish that, he has introduced into his picture of brain processes his own premises about human nature. The inevitability of doing precisely that in no way mitigates its significance in Young's case. Brains cannot be isolated from persons any more than persons can be isolated from brains.

## Mental Phenomena and the Brain

The "mind-body problem" concerns the way we think about states of consciousness on one hand and states of behavior on the other. What is the interaction between thoughts, feelings and the organ responsible for their expression, the brain? The problem, at heart, is how to hold together the *obvious* characteristics of people and their external behavior, and the not-so-obvious characteristics such as their internal mental states. Often the dilemma is expressed as the tension between the material and the immaterial, between brain and mind, between body and soul. Thought, feelings and beliefs are frequently described as constituting the mind; with increasing comprehension of brain mechanisms, however, they may seem to be products of physical brain processes rather than, or at least as much as, of an immaterial mind or spirit.

Although the mind-body problem is an old issue in philosophy, advances in the neurosciences over the past twenty or thirty years have forced the neuropsychologist to deal with it also. Many of the topics we have discussed, especially the split-brain studies and the brain-damage/personality paradigm, highlight the problem in a new way. Whether they help solve that longstanding dilemma is debatable.

The mind-body problem forces neuroscientists to consider not only their philosophical position on that question but also the nature of their science. Inevitably neuroscientists start from their knowledge of the brain as a physical entity or of the individual as a group of observable behavior patterns. Once confronted by the possible existence of an immaterial mind, neuroscientists must assess the adequacy of their observable base of physical phenomena. They must ask whether it alone provides an all-embracing framework for a complete view of the individual person as a human being like themselves. By the very nature of the scientific endeavor, neuroscientists may find themselves drawn toward some form of materialist answer without analyzing the philosophical implications of such an answer.

Let us briefly review the major positions that have developed in the debate, starting inevitably with René Descartes and *dualism*. Descartes, as we saw in chapter 1, devoted some thought to neurobiological considerations along with his better known mathematical and philosophical studies. Living at a time when the natural sciences were being revolutionized by mechanistic thinking, Descartes compared the universe to a vast machine capable of being explained by purely mechanical laws. Everything, including man himself, was encompassed by these all-powerful explanatory principles. In arguing thus, Descartes was being true to his rationalism. Yet, unable to follow rationalism to its logical conclusion, he allowed one exception to his mechanical world view: the human mind.

Descartes, intent on doubting the evidence of the senses and calling into question even the validity of his perceptions of the world, felt able to fall back on the trustworthiness of his own consciousness. Hence the fundamental divide within dualism between the *physical body* and the *nonphysical mind* or consciousness, the former a prisoner of the mechanical world-order but the latter the author of uniquely human characteristics such as rational thought and free choice. For Descartes it was the nonphysical mind which rendered a human being unique and which carried the marks of personhood. That nonphysical side of humans—the mind, soul or consciousness—was the critical one, constituting, alongside the body, one of the two basic *substances* of the world.

The essence of classic dualism is the existence of body and mind as distinct substances. They were regarded by Descartes as totally interdependent, interacting aspects of a living being. If that is so, however, the way in which they interact becomes a problem. According to Descartes, the mind took up no space but acted on the body through the brain's pineal gland. The nonmaterial mind could thus influence physical happenings in the material brain. The hallmark of this view, *interactionism,* is the implicit suggestion that two different types of reality can affect one another.

Cartesian dualism was little challenged from Descartes's time in the seventeenth century until the late nineteenth century. The inherent difficulty of two different substances acting on each other, however, led some dualists to adopt an aberrant version of dualism, called *parallelism:* the mind and body are still distinct, but run along parallel tracks. To declare them independent proved a convenient way out of the interactionist dilemma, but opened the window to an influx of weird speculation. Without any control of each other, body and mind could go their own ways even to the extent of dispensing with the material body altogether.

We shall return to dualism in the next section when considering the viewpoint of contemporary neurophysiologist John Eccles. But before leaving dualism we should note one reason for its continuing influence up to the end of the last century and, in some quarters, up to the present: it seemed to offer support for the Christian belief in an immortal soul. Reflecting the Platonic concept of the soul, the classical form of that belief was strongly dualistic. A danger of dualism, however, is that once body and mind are separated, the mind can be dealt with as a separate entity. A modern consequence of dualism is that drug-induced perceptions and beliefs can be regarded as a valid—even a commendable—expression of reality. John Lilly, whose views we explored in the previous chapter is a modern exponent of parallelism. A perennial danger of that outlook is that the exaltation of mind takes place at the expense of the whole person.

The major difficulty with dualism is the unknowability of internal mental states if we have no way of analyzing them by way of behavioral or brain states. If mental states are not publicly observable, we cannot even be sure that we are justified in ascribing them to other people at all. The chasm between unknown internal states and known external ones makes information on how mental and brain states are to be linked difficult (some would say impossible) to obtain. It is far from clear whether any links between the two are of a causal nature; hence the possibility of parallelism.

The difficulties associated with dualism have led to an array of alternative positions. The first alternative is, strictly speaking, a version of dualism with similarities to parallelism. In *epiphenomenalism,* a nonmaterial mind is considered to exist but is an epiphenomenon or byproduct of physical events. Consequently, the conscious events of the mind are unable to influence the physical brain and its processes. The thoughts, moods and decisions of an individual, therefore, are powerless to influence that individual's actions.

Epiphenomenalism, like classic dualism, accepts an immaterial mind. On the other hand, like materialism, it locates the origin of mind in the material brain. It is a compromise that seems to exhibit the difficulties of both positions without satisfying exponents of either. The contention of epiphenomenalism that consciousness has no effect on the way the brain operates makes a mockery of human beliefs, actions and conscious choices. For anyone with a high view of the human person and human brain, epiphenomenalism is unsatisfactory.

A more rigorous alternative to dualism is *behaviorism,* which attempts to eliminate nonphysical mental states altogether by reducing them to patterns of behavior. That form of behaviorism is sometimes referred to as *negative* behaviorism, signifying that it is essentially a metaphysical doctrine rather than a straightforward psychological technique.

For a behaviorist, any talk about a mind is simply an inaccurate way of talking about human behavior. It is a form of linguistic confusion because the mind is neither a thing nor a substance, in the way the brain is a thing. Only the brain can be referred to in these terms; such terminology is inappropriate when referring to actions, thoughts, feelings and desires. If they are expressions of brain states, they are best described and analyzed using behavioral concepts.

We have already discussed the demise of the mind within a Skinnerian framework. By denigrating individual consciousness, behaviorism is driven to look for forces controlling individual behavior either in the physiological makeup of the individual or in that person's environment; hence the significance of conditioning as a technology of behavior. Since individuals are merely the sum of their behavior patterns, behaviorism has dispensed not only with consciousness and internal mental states but also with human freedom, human dignity and human responsibility.

On the surface, behaviorism, with its simple reduction of mental states to actual or potential behavior, seems a welcome contrast to the tantalizing complexities of dualism. Yet its pitfalls are immense. The argument that all reference to the mind is simply a prescientific description of states of behavior is misleading. To say that "to be angry" means to behave in an angry way overlooks the possibility that someone may be angry but not show it. Further, the statement by itself explains nothing: angry behavior is angry behavior. Another difficulty is that we frequently appear to know more about our own mental states than other people do—a contradiction in terms if our mental states are nothing but patterns of behavior.

That mental states can, to some extent, be analyzed in behavioral terms is not open to question; that they can be *completely* analyzed in that manner, is. If they cannot be completely analyzed in behavioral terms, the issue of the nature of mental states remains. Apart from that dilemma, however, behaviorism can definitely be faulted for its loss of the wholeness and grandeur of the human person.

A third alternative to dualism is based on the presupposition that mental states are identical with brain states. The mind-brain identity theory is called *central-state material-*

*ism.* In its simplest expression it asserts that the goings-on in the mind are manifestations of physical happenings within the brain. Unlike behaviorism, it makes no attempt to deny the existence of consciousness or mental events; they are realities, but of the material brain rather than of an immaterial mind.

To equate the mind with the brain bypasses certain difficulties evident in epiphenomenalism and behaviorism. The self-evident phenomenon of consciousness is retained, and the problem of explaining how mind and brain interact does not arise. Central-state materialism has many attractive features to anyone aware of the dependence of conscious states on brain function.

Nevertheless, it too has its drawbacks. It is easy to assert a oneness of the mind and brain but much more difficult to demonstrate what that identity amounts to specifically. As discussed earlier, J. Z. Young's attempt to do that necessitated a leap of faith to help bridge the gap between brain mechanisms and the meaning of human life. Such a leap may be tantamount to admitting that even if mind and brain processes are not identical, at the very least they provide clues to different aspects of human reality.

If one assumes that mind and brain are identical, what are the implications of that outlook for our view of human nature? Does it threaten the concept of human freedom by necessitating belief in determinism? In other words, acceptance of the validity of materialism precipitates a new discussion—that of determinism. We shall address that issue shortly.

Neither dualism nor any of its alternatives provide a fully satisfying solution to the brain-mind controversy. Each illustrates some truth about the human person and human brain, yet each fails to hold the available data and insights in a manageable form. We would be tempted to dismiss all philosophical speculation and settle for a formula solution if the stakes were not so high. With the dignity and worth of human beings in the balance, some way forward must be found.

## Contemporary Dualism

From the preceding discussion one might conclude that dualism has fallen into such disrepute that no respectable philosopher—certainly no respectable neurobiologist—would give it serious consideration as being of anything but historical interest. Yet dualism has been propounded in its classic form for at least twenty years by a respected and notable neurophysiologist, Sir John Eccles. What is more, his advocacy has become increasingly firm and vigorous over the years, coming to full fruition in the 1970s. Eccles leans heavily on the writings of Sir Karl Popper, particularly on the ideas expressed in Popper's three-world philosophy. The interaction between Popper the philosopher and Eccles the neurobiologist resulted in a joint magnum opus, *The Self and Its Brain,* lauding dualism and interactionism. Eccles has expressed his views in many speeches, articles and books, including the 1977-78 Gifford Lectures at the University of Edinburgh, published as *The Human Mystery.*

Eccles's enthusiasm for dualism appears to go back to another great neurophysiologist, Sir Charles Sherrington, whose own Gifford Lectures on the theme *Man on His Nature* were published in 1940. Sherrington was a dualist who felt the pangs of disconnectedness between brain and mind but found no answer to the dilemma of how the two cohere. Eccles also recognizes dualist aspirations in the writings of more recent scientists, notably physicists Erwin Schrö-dinger and Eugene Wigner and ethologist W. H. Thorpe. Underlying the views of such thinkers is the primacy of our conscious experiences, which constitute for us primary or first-order reality. By contrast, the so-called objective or material world is a derivative or second-order reality. The world around us is known to exist only because *we* experience it. We are in a position to describe and understand the world only on account of our self-consciousness, which is another way of saying that our minds are primary in knowing.

Emphasis on the primacy of consciousness does not inevitably lead to the strident dualism advocated by Eccles.

As we shall see in the next section, it forms the starting point of Donald MacKay's alternative notion of logical indeterminacy. For Eccles, however, the primacy of consciousness leads to a dualism diametrically opposed to what he describes as monist-materialism. The latter he sees as ushering in a world of chance and circumstance, with no meaning for life, no values, no freedom and no responsibility. Against this, he wishes to put forward a world view incorporating the mystery of our existence, its supernatural meaning and the fact that we are part of some great design. Beside being a dualist, therefore, Eccles is also a finalist, believing that our individual lives have a role to play in some great unimaginable supernatural drama.

The motives of Eccles and Popper are, from a Christian perspective, exemplary. They are intent on viewing human beings as ends in themselves, with meaning, values, purpose and responsibility. In starting from the self-consciousness of individuals, they insure that individuals will not be reduced to partial materialistic components and thereby lose their personhood. For such strong premises we are grateful. But when Eccles and Popper proceed beyond basic principles there is cause for concern. Their defense of human dignity and meaning rests on an explicit dualism between the self and the brain; the self-conscious mind is described as acting on the neural centers of the brain, thereby modifying the dynamic spatio-temporal patterns of the neural events. If such *interactionism* par excellence should fail as an explanatory principle, human dignity and meaning are placed in serious jeopardy. The issue is not simply whether dualism and interactionism can be justified, therefore, but whether this is an appropriate way to defend human significance.

Karl Popper's three-world view, developed in the early 1970s, is depicted in Figure 8.1. *World 1* is the world of physical objects and states. It comprises, therefore, inorganic matter, the whole of biology and the material substratum of all manmade artefacts. *World 2* is the realm of states

*Figure 8.1   Three-world view of Popper. Adapted from K. R. Popper and J. C. Eccles, The Self and Its Brain, © 1977. Used by permission of Springer-Verlag.*

| World 1 | World 2 | World 3 |
|---|---|---|
| Physical objects and states | States of consciousness | Knowledge in objective sense |
| 1. Inorganic Matter and energy of cosmos | Subjective knowledge | Cultural heritage coded on material substrates |
| 2. Biology Structure and actions of all living beings —human brains | Experience of perception thinking emotions dispositional intentions memories dreams creative imagination | philosophical theological scientific historical literary artistic technological |
| 3. Artefacts Material substrates of human creativity of tools of machines of books of works of art of music | | Theoretical systems scientific problems critical arguments |

of consciousness; it is the world each of us knows firsthand, containing our ongoing experiences of perception, thinking, emotions, imaginings and memories. Of particular significance in Popper's philosophical scheme is *World 3,* the world of knowledge in the objective sense. Encompassed by that world are all the records of human culture expressed in scientific, literary and artistic thoughts, plus the theoretical systems comprising scientific problems and the critical arguments generated by the discussion of those problems. World 3 is the world of human intellectual endeavor, a world of culture and storage.

The uniqueness of man, according to Eccles, is that he not only exists in World 1, the world of matter and energy, but can also realize his existence in World 2, the world of self-awareness. It is their World 2 existence that bestows a soul on human beings. Human experience does not stop at World 2, however, because human beings utilize their World 2 knowledge to create yet another world, that of culture (World 3). In that third world human greatness manifests itself with the rise of cultures and civilizations. What we are is dependent on World 3 in which we have been immersed and on the effectiveness with which we have utilized our opportunities to make the most of our brain potentialities.

At the level of the individual, Eccles argues that the brain in World 1 and the world of culture in World 3 are both necessary for the development of the conscious self in World 2 (Fig. 8.1). Eccles goes beyond expression of the three-world view, however, to contend that such interaction is not sufficient to explain the uniqueness of our personal self. The explanation must lie outside the field of scientific inquiry; the

*Figure 8.2  Information flow diagram for brain-mind interaction, as postulated by Eccles. Adapted from J. C. Eccles,* Facing Reality, *©1970. Used by permission of Springer-Verlag and the author.*

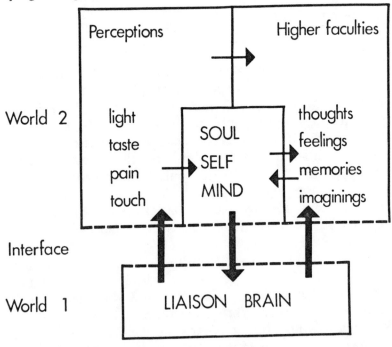

coming-into-existence of each unique self is the result of a supernatural creation of the soul.

In taking up that position, Eccles has already committed himself to a strong dualist position on the brain-mind problem. He regards brain and mind as independent entities, with the brain in World 1 and the mind in World 2 (Fig. 8.1). What is more, they are thought to interact, as outlined in Figure 8.2, across the World 1-World 2 interface. Eccles concludes that the world of matter and energy, including the brain (World 1), is not completely sealed off from the world of experience and subjective experiences (the mind, World 2). Their interaction allows the mind to influence the brain or, more specifically, the self-conscious mind to influence the neuronal machinery of the brain.

In working out his position, Eccles postulates that the self-conscious mind influences neural events in special areas of the neocortex which he terms the *liaison brain*. These areas can perhaps be compared to the pineal gland in Descartes's scheme of things. To substantiate a dualist-interactionist view, there must be loopholes or crevices in World 1 (the brain) enabling it to be modified by World 2 (conscious experience). Eccles's loopholes are provided by the liaison brain (Fig. 8.2).

Two issues immediately arise. Is it the mind or the brain that is responsible for the unity of conscious experience? What is the evidence for the existence of a liaison brain?

Eccles categorically asserts that the unity of conscious experience is provided by the self-conscious mind and not by the neuronal machinery of the liaison brain. His reason appears to be the inadequacy of any neurophysiological theory in that regard. Eccles rejects the notion that the self-conscious mind is in liaison with single nerve cells, contending instead that liaison occurs with groups of nerve cells in the cerebral cortex known as modules. The liaison modules are found principally in the dominant left hemisphere, particularly the linguistic areas, because in split-brain subjects, consciousness is principally located in the left hemisphere with its speech centers. The prefrontal lobe of the dominant hemisphere is also, in Eccles's eyes, a highly probable liaison site, since memory storage and retrieval may be located there. A brain-mind interactionist position is also suggested, Eccles claims, by physiological evidence of a readiness potential and by work on the subjective correlates of cortical stimulation.

The details of these arguments are beyond the scope of this book, but they are all open to alternative interpretations by neurophysiologists. The areas of the cerebral-hemisphere-designated liaison areas have no morphologically distinguishing features from nonliaison areas. It must be admitted that since no one has any idea what to look for, a scientific approach is valueless at present. But that is precisely the difficulty with the liaison brain concept: it expresses in semiscientific language an idea that is essentially ascientific. It must be questioned, therefore, whether the "liaison brain" really does belong to World 1, as Eccles suggests—or to World 2.

How successful has Eccles been in reinterpreting Cartesian dualism in contemporary neuroscientific terms? More important, does he provide grounds for recommending such strong dualism to Christians? Has he given us an alternative to materialistic monism?

Excellent as his intentions are, it is doubtful that Eccles has succeeded in his quest. The inevitably debatable nature of his neurophysiological interpretations is reminiscent of the constantly recurring "God-of-the-gaps" syndrome. The interface between the mind/self/soul and the brain shifts from one brain region or set of nerve cells to another as the scientific evidence and its interpretation shift. There is no escape from that dilemma, as long as one is dealing with the scientific domain. Eccles, who once staked his claim for an interface in the synapse, is now prepared to stake it elsewhere. Any specific location must, by the nature of the situation, prove temporary.

The fundamental problem of dualism is the feasibility of

one sort of substance acting on another sort of substance. If the mind/self/soul acts on modules of nerve cells as modules act on each other, is the mind/self/soul something like a module? Alternatively, if the mind/self/soul acts in an inexplicable way, does it become an inexplicable entity? That is where Descartes had to leave the problem. In spite of Eccles's detailed neurophysiological postulates, the mind remains inexplicable and the way it interacts with the brain is a pseudoexplanation in Eccles's system. If the mind is nonphysical, can it have a physical interaction with the brain? If its interaction is nonphysical, does it then become a nonproblem for neuroscientists?

The brain is subject to scientific scrutiny because it is publicly observable; the mind or soul is not open to such investigation and hence can never receive scientific support. Proof that the mind or soul either is or is not influencing the brain is almost impossible to obtain. Either way, it needs to be demonstrated that the brain does or does not possess some device for receiving influences from the mind. Eccles attempts to demonstrate that such a device does exist, bringing us back to the equivocal status of the whole exercise. On the other hand, there is ample evidence that human behavior is caused by neural events; the evidence that every neural event is caused by some physical event is not conclusive, but neither can it be ignored.

A final difficulty with the strong dualism of Eccles and Popper is perhaps surprising. The fact is that radical dualism is in danger of overlooking the human person. It tries to uphold the meaning of human existence not so much at the personal level as at the level of brain-mind interaction. True, Eccles uses as his starting point our awareness of our conscious selves. But that awareness becomes lost amid his neuroscientific justification of how and where the self-conscious mind exerts its control over the brain. It may be that any emphasis on the separation of brain and mind, of body and soul, misses the crucial, intimate relationship *we,* as people, have to our bodies. The form of dualism advocated by Eccles may simply be misplaced.

Before leaving contemporary dualism we should consider two other examples from the ranks of neuroscientists. Wilder Penfield, one of the most influential neurosurgeons of this century, made major contributions to the localization of function in the cerebral hemispheres in the 1930s and '40s (see chapter 1). Like Eccles, Penfield was influenced by Sherrington's ideas on the relationship between the brain and mind, but an explicitly dualistic position emerged only gradually throughout his long life. Penfield's dualism is expressed most clearly in *The Mystery of the Mind,* published in 1975 when he was eighty-five years old.

For Penfield the mind is aware of what is going on, it focuses attention, reasons and makes decisions, but has no memory of its own. It can put decisions into effect by activating nerve cell mechanisms situated in what Penfield terms the highest brain-mechanism, a region of grey matter in the upper reaches of the brain stem. The highest brain-mechanism, therefore, functions as the messenger between the mind and other brain-mechanisms. It serves as the mind's executive, its normal action constituting the physical basis of the mind.

Penfield was drawn to his view by his experience with patients displaying a variety of brain lesions. In particular he was impressed by attacks of epileptic automatism, in which a patient becomes unconscious but continues to act as an automaton. Penfield recognized in that situation a dissociation between the functions of the automatic sensory-motor mechanism and the highest brain-mechanism. He surmised that the highest brain-mechanism might go out of action during such attacks, depriving the patient of the functions of the mind.

For Penfield, as for Eccles, belief in a distinct and purposeful mind proved a buttress against the inroads of materialism. Its mystery intrigued him, and even if we find his arguments unconvincing, it is hard to escape the sense of the wonder at human thought and the complexity of the neural machinery that comes through in his writings. His awe at the potential of the human intellect and the subtleties of behavior of a brain-damaged patient demands a serious response on our part.

R. W. Sperry appeared in chapter 2 as one of the foremost exponents of split-brain studies. Sperry has also written extensively in the brain-mind area. Although not a dualist in the classic sense exemplified by Eccles and Penfield, he fits best within that general category.

Like Eccles and Penfield, Sperry wants to reject both behaviorism and materialism. More specifically, he rejects theories of consciousness that interpret subjective experience as an epiphenomenon, or parallel correlate of brain activity, or as identical to neural events.

Sperry advocates a form of *emergence*, in which consciousness is an emergent property of brain activity. Conscious phenomena are different from, more than, and not reducible to neural events, although they are built of neural and other physicochemical events. He sees value in a description of the neural events generating conscious experience, while denying that such a description can arrive at a complete understanding of consciousness. Most important within Sperry's system is his view that the emergent properties forming the mind are capable of controlling normal brain processes.

Sperry, recognizing that no direct empirical proof exists, argues that his position is more credible than the behaviorist-materialist position. The difference between himself and Eccles is in the absence of a specific dualist interaction in Sperry's system. Instead, conscious experience influences the brain by virtue of the hierarchical organization of the nervous system and in the power exerted by a whole over its parts. From Sperry's perspective, mind moves matter in the brain in much the same way that an organism moves its component organs and cells.

Sperry leans heavily on the role played by subjective conscious experience in an appreciation of brain function. The significance of that role, in his eyes, is that the value-rich, qualitative world of inner, conscious, subjective experience is reinstated into the domain of science. He is thus able to introduce into neuroscience what he calls humanistic thinking, leading to an erasure of the distinction between objective facts and subjective values.

Sperry's approach to the brain-mind issue, therefore, is part of a much broader issue—that of introducing values into science. Intent on deriving an ethical framework from science, Sperry sets about demonstrating that human values are inherent properties of brain activity and hence amenable to scientific investigation. That assumption leads him to propose a value system built on the orderly design of evolving nature.

Sperry's view seems to be a curious amalgam of materialism and dualism. Although he claims to be strongly anti-materialist, the emergent mind of his scheme is entirely a product of neural events. Once mind has emerged, however, it assumes the dominant role in driving the brain, being the essential directive force of brain processes. The mind is seen as being above the brain processes even though they are described as mutually interdependent. Since Sperry's holism arises from material forces *within* the brain, his stance—unlike that of Eccles—is thoroughly antisupernatural. If an emergent scheme is eclectic, allowing arbitrary values to be introduced into it, it seems to provide no surer way to a humane society than materialism.

Another difficulty with emergence reflects its dualistic leanings. Even if conscious experience does emerge from neural organization, the mode of control then exercised by consciousness remains unexplained. Either we are back at the interaction problem, or consciousness adds nothing to the wholeness generated by the brain itself.

In the end we are not fully satisfied with Sperry's position, although we agree on the importance of subjective conscious experience. A longing for holism is exemplary, but Sperry's rejection of a Christian outlook limits his horizons to the materialism that so distresses him. What Sperry has overlooked is the contribution that can be made by adopting more than one perspective to the wholeness of the human person. The brain-mind blem, like the science-values issue, should be viewed from different viewpoints. When that is done, previously unrecognized aspects may appear. It is to such a "perspectivalist" approach that we now turn.

## Brains and Persons

Dualists take subjective experience seriously but sometimes stumble over its implications. Brain scientist Donald Mac-Kay suggests that we start from our immediate experience of what it is like to be a person. Our primary data constitute a flood of conscious experiences such as seeing, hearing, thinking, meeting people. Taken together, these data form the ground on which *all* our knowledge must rest. Alongside these data one also has other characteristics, so that being a person means being identifiable to other persons as a tangible body and having specific conscious experiences like those of other persons.

MacKay sees in that description of a person a dualism of *two different kinds of data* about ourselves. There are data of our own experience as conscious agents, and data about our correlated brain activity and brain states. Put more simply, the first is the *I-story,* what we see and believe; the second is the *brain-story,* the corresponding processes going on within our brains. Every aspect of our conscious experience, anything we believe or see or hear, will be represented by a particular configuration in the state of our brains. From that it follows that a *change* in our experience will be accompanied by a *change* in the state of our brains. This is a basic assumption of brain science, although we still know very little about the actual organization of the brain under changing circumstances.

If we accept that assumption for the purpose of argument, what follows from it? It has often been suggested that the two must be *causally* related, that is, the I-story must cause the brain-story or vice versa. MacKay's contribution comes in at just that point. He does not deny that such a causal connection may occur, but contends that it is implausible and unnecessary.

Instead of viewing the two sets of events as rivals, so that one must be right and the other wrong, MacKay suggests that we view them as *complementary* aspects of human behavior. "These events," he writes, "admit of analysis at the mechanical level in terms of nerve cells and their interactions, and also not only admit of but demand analysis in terms of their significance as the activity of a conscious being whose thoughts and desires and decisions can determine his behaviour."

Taking his argument further, MacKay tackles the problem of determinism. If a "superscientist" were able to specify every aspect of the machinery of an individual's brain, would that individual be correct to believe all the specifications he was told about the state of his brain? In other words, may a point be reached one day when by analyzing an individual's brain a scientist would be able to tell that individual what he would believe at some future time? Or, to be more exact, what he would be *correct* to believe? If so, freedom of action and responsibility would become mere illusions.

MacKay contends there is a logical fallacy in that argument. If an individual were to believe what he was told about the state of his brain, his belief would have a major consequence: the state of his brain would be immediately changed by introduction of that new (belief) factor. Therefore, he would be *mistaken* to believe what he was told, because that description would be out of date. Thus no complete specification of a brain's mechanism can exist which would be equally correct whether or not the person concerned believed it. The point of the argument is that an observer's prediction would be valid only if he did *not* inform the individual being observed of his prediction.

Could the time ever come when allowance can also be made for the new factor? MacKay says no: even if it becomes possible to produce a specification which is incorrect at the moment but will *become* correct when it is believed, there would still be a difficulty. The difficulty is that the individual concerned would be under no obligation actually to believe it. If he did believe it, it would be correct; but if he did not believe it, it would be incorrect. And there is no reason why he should believe it. Consequently, MacKay contends, there can never be produced a specification of a person's brain, however sophisticated, that would have an *unconditional* claim to his assent.

The consequence is that, even if the human brain turns out to be as mechanical as the solar system, predictions about it will always differ from predictions about the solar system. Although predictions about the latter may have an unconditional claim to our assent, predictions about our brains do not—because we are under no obligation to believe them. The future state of our brains is *indeterminate* for us until we have decided on a course of action or belief. It is indeterminate not just in the sense of being unknown, but because a future specification does not exist which is inevitable for us until we have made up our minds.

MacKay argues that there are thus no mechanistic grounds for excusing our actions. We *are* responsible beings. MacKay spells out the crux of that responsibility, decision making. "A decision," he says, "is an action whose future form depends on what you believe about the situation in a way that makes it *indeterminate for you* until you have made up your mind: indeterminate, not just in the sense of *unknown* to you, but in the sense that there does not exist a specification of the outcome which is *inevitable* for you until you make up your mind: until, in other words, you determine what the form shall be."

Human decision making provides a basis of freedom for us —even in a mechanistic universe. We are free and responsible, not in spite of the way our brains work or because of the way our brains work, but because freedom of action is a demonstrable, logical fact. MacKay's principle of *logical indeterminacy* applies even in a physically determinate universe, although of course it is far from certain that the universe is in fact physically determinate. MacKay's point is that, even if such an extreme situation were to prevail, his principle would continue to hold.

A crucial point for MacKay's stance is that the I-story (mind-story) and the brain-story are *correlates* of one another and not translations of one another. That means that the I-story can be indeterministic and the brain-story deterministic without mutual contradiction. The reason is that the two statements are descriptions of different aspects of an event, one referring to people with brains and the other to the brains of people. When considering the question of freedom, it is important to distinguish between people and brains—because it is people, and not brains, who are free. Conversely, it is brains, and not people, which may be machines.

MacKay's concern throughout is to demonstrate that any denial of human responsibility on the basis of the assumed physical determinateness of the brain is based on a *logical* error. Hence the positive scientific theory that all physical events are determined by physical causes does not, he argues, imply the negative metaphysical belief that the immediate future of a human agent is inevitable. It follows that, even if an individual's action is predictable by observers, there would be no ground for denying that individual's responsibility for it.

It is evident that MacKay, unlike Eccles, does not seek gaps in physical causality within the brain. Conscious activity is embodied in the brain activity that physically determines what our bodies do. The mental and the physical are in no sense rivals, therefore, but are complementary aspects of our consciousness. Beside the primacy of conscious experience, MacKay stresses the necessity to attach the significance of human identity to a person as a whole rather than to an artificially isolated body or brain.

MacKay's defense of human freedom on the basis of logical indeterminacy has attracted the attention of many philosophers. If legitimate, it provides a means of circumventing the seemingly intractable problems of dualism and the potentially dehumanizing tendencies of materialism.

A major question posed by MacKay's argument is the meaning of the term *freedom*. Stephen Evans, in his book *Preserving the Person*, considers that MacKay's argument can be interpreted in two ways. According to the first, an individual is free as long as he is kept in ignorance of the observer's predictions about his future actions. The individual is free in the sense that he has alternatives he could choose if different conditions prevailed. In that instance, the freedom of the individual lies in his lack of knowledge of the particular prediction made by the observer. The second interpretation entails a more rigorous meaning of freedom, namely, that no logical specifications exist of an individual's beliefs about a subject on which he is at present undecided. An individual's future belief is indeterminate, since any prediction about that belief might change it. Believing is not merely a physical happening, therefore; it includes a normative element about what *ought* to be believed. If that is true, an individual reflecting on the causes of his beliefs may proceed to alter those beliefs, the implication being that beliefs are not just events to be causally determined and predicted. They result from rational reflection and hence may be free because of the nature of such reflection. If so, an onlooker as well as the individual may agree that beliefs of that type are free.

Evans favors the second alternative interpretation of MacKay's argument as a basis for human freedom. Both the potential strengths and weaknesses of MacKay's position seem to lie in its purely logical level. Although MacKay demonstrates the pitfalls of materialism and points the way to a viable alternative to both it and dualism, many find his argument hard to follow. The meaning of freedom may be one issue that needs clarification. It is clear that MacKay believes that freedom is real and not an illusion.

MacKay appears to be saying that, if a future outcome is

indeterminate for an individual, that individual has the power to determine the outcome, and therefore is free. Freedom of that kind underlies human responsibility. MacKay has put forward a very strong argument that there are future beliefs that are *indeterminate for* the individual. What is less clear is whether this implies that such beliefs are *determinable by* the individual.

MacKay's logical argument fits well with his Christian presuppositions. It is a clearing operation for working out the meaning and consequences of belief in human freedom and dignity. MacKay has shown that man cannot be written off as a being for whom all future thoughts, actions and decisions are inevitable. Having established that, the task is now to demonstrate what human freedom entails and the uses to which it needs to be put.

In a sense, our discussion has brought us a long way from the brain-mind debate. Yet the direction we have traveled has been almost an inevitable one for a Christian. We dare not isolate a person's brain from the remainder of the body and personality as though it were a detachable piece of luggage. To reach a person-centered conclusion one must start from *man as a person,* not from man as a brain.

Many discussions of brain-mind relationships bypass a holistic view of human beings, then find it impossible to break free of the bonds of reductionism. To confine one's perspective of the mind to specific regions of the brain demeans the value of human significance, regardless of the conclusions reached. A proper level at which to contemplate the brain-mind debate is that of humans as choosing, deliberating, valuing and purposeful beings. From that vantage point, the primacy of our own consciousness is a valid piece of evidence. Our sense of freedom and purpose is an essential ingredient of any discussion on the human brain and what has traditionally been termed the human mind.

## Human Dignity and Human Aspirations
To start with men and women as beings aware of their own

and other people's consciousness may appear to circumvent some of the traditional difficulties simply by ignoring them. Yet that starting point may also lead to exploration of new dimensions of insight, as it seems to do in MacKay's thinking. Many challenges arising from the application of brain research are challenges to the integrity of the human person. We must see the brain in the context of the value of the human person.

In chapter 2 we were confronted with the meaning of humanness in biological terms. The characteristics emerging there included an awareness of oneself as an individual, understanding of oneself and one's goals, ability to judge oneself and others, self-reflection, creativity and awareness of one's own transcience. Perhaps the supreme characteristic of humanness, beyond the narrowly biological, is our potential for responding to the overtures of God. That potential implies that we are beings stemming from the purposes of God and achieving significance and freedom within the designs of God.

Compartmentalization is an ever-present danger. Human beings are both biological and spiritual beings. There is nothing wrong with those two designations but only with the idea that one part of human nature is biological and another part spiritual. When that idea surfaces, we are back at "interactionism." Of course, at the whole-person level, the parallel of brain-mind dualism is body-soul dualism. Compartmentalization gives us human beings made up of a body plus a soul, a material entity plus an immaterial entity.

In place of that type of dualism we must contend for the holism of the human person. Each person is a unity describable as a biological-spiritual being, as a body-soul, or as a material-immaterial entity. For certain purposes a person can usefully be compared to a machine. But he is simultaneously and equally a person created by God, not one more than the other. The fact that persons are one of those reflects the fact that they are also the other; they cannot be simply one without the other. Both facets of their being are necessary for them to be human. The two complementary descriptions are intimately interwoven aspects of what being human is all about.

Once the unitary vision of a human being is grasped, we are unlikly to be satisfied with any one-sided analysis of human significance. Nor can we be satisfied with an overtly compartmentalized view of the human condition. In contrast to the Gnostic view of matter as inherently evil, the Bible affirms the goodness of the created order and hence of matter. Yet to limit human horizons to matter is a gross denial of our relationship to God and our grounding in the purposes of God. Even an intermediate position that fears a mechanistic description of man is inadequate if it unduly elevates human spirituality.

Each person as a unity transcending the vistas of the observable, yet thoroughly biological, is the principal position to which we wish to cling. That view appears both to express the essence of the biblical teaching and to provide a meaningful way to approach contemporary neurobiology.

Turning first to Scripture, we find different terms used by Old and New Testament writers to refer to body, soul, spirit and heart, but the unity of the human person is the underlying theme throughout the Bible. Much of the time and effort expended on distinguishing the precise connotations of these terms has seemed to dismantle the person into discrete segments.

Although the biblical writers found it convenient to view man as consisting of different elements, there is no hint of a mere parallelism between the two predominant elements, body and soul. That dichotomy, so beloved in Greek philosophy, is foreign to the Bible, in which every human act is seen as the act of the whole person. Louis Berkhof in his *Systematic Theology* says: "It is not the soul but man that sins; it is not the body but man that dies; and it is not merely the soul, but man, body and soul, that is redeemed in Christ." The idea of unity is brought out clearly in the Genesis account of man's creation by God, in which we are told that God formed man from the dust of the ground and breathed into his nostrils the breath of life. The result was that man became a living creature, or as the King James version phrases it, a living soul. The soul *(nephesh)* of that translation means a living being; life bound up with a body, the sort of life shared also by animals. In the Genesis account, it is *man* who came into being, not his body alone or any other segment of him.

Throughout the Old Testament, the emphasis is always on the whole life of a person, never on a body as the material element and a soul as the spiritual element. Biblical Hebrew, lacking a word for the body as an organism, distinguished between higher and lower elements within human nature. The higher elements are represented by words such as spirit, soul, heart and mind; the lower by flesh, dust, bones, bowels and kidneys. The most important organ within that range is heart, denoting the whole personality, the intellect, the will or the emotions. The biblical "heart," therefore, covering a diversity of physical, emotional and rational functions, helps to illustrate man's unity as a complex body-mind-spirit-soul entity.

The New Testament concept of the person is more tortuous to unravel because of its use of the Greek language and, inevitably, certain Greek modes of thought. Several words are used interchangeably to refer to the whole person. These Greek words, including the ones commonly translated as soul, body, spirit and flesh, characterize various aspects of the life and relationships of the person. For example, *pneuma* (spirit) denotes a person's relationship with God, while *sarx* (flesh) points to a person's alienation from God. Those terms do not support a conception of human beings as possessing a soullike entity. They signify rather the quality of the life of a person in relation to God and other human beings.

Although it may be difficult to reconcile some passages of Scripture with a unitary view of the human person, there can be little doubt that *wholeness* is the mark of the biblical attitude. Fragmentation into distinct substances is not part of the biblical framework.

The principal repercussion of the biblical view is a discarding of the Greek idea of an "immortal soul." What is stressed is not the immortality of the soul (and dissolution of the body) at death, but the Christian hope that God will reconstitute the *whole* person. The picture painted by the apostle Paul in 1 Corinthians 15 is of a perfect, imperishable, glorious resurrected body which, for want of a better term, he calls a "spiritual body." Words fail in this area, but Paul's emphasis on wholeness comes through when he likens Christians after death to the "heavenly man," Jesus Christ himself. For Paul, the ultimate hope for Christians is that we will experience a wholeness and completeness inaccessible to us in this life. All that we are now will be transformed, so that we will know a total renewal of our body-mind unit.

The Christian hope is a far cry from an afterlife inhabited by ethereal, disembodied souls. It is also a far cry from philosophical edifices constructed on psychical phenomena, on "out of the body" experiences accompanying resuscitation after clinical death or on the use of psychedelic drugs (chapter 7). Whatever one's interpretation of these phenomena, they need to be seen against the background of pervasive belief in an immortal soul. In the circumstances under which the phenomena occur, with the brain itself probably generating hallucinations, the resulting experiences seem to confirm the underlying premise. Radical separation between the brain and mind is part of that premise, with the mind engaging in activities and creative adventures in isolation from the brain and body. Implicit within all such fantasies is a fragmentation of the person, a step on the road to the disintegration of the personality.

The wholeness of the human person advocated here allows no sharp distinction between brain and mind, the brain being the *basis* of all that we know of the personality in this life. To understand human beings as persons is to accept them for what they are, to encourage the development of interrelationships with other people and with God, and to provide opportunities for them to exercise choices and make decisions. Human beings are characterized by what they are and can do as conscious agents. For this their brains are essential, yet an understanding of brains as neural machines is not the way to a complete understanding of human beings as persons. The level of explanation is inappropriate. Human beings are not simply neural machines clothed with bodies, but living creatures with goals, purposes, aspirations, hopes, fears and self-awareness, who have been created to respond to God and to delight in him and his purposes and aspirations.

Although mind is a term traditionally employed to cover the mental abilities of human beings, it is not always a helpful concept. Instead, one can emphasize personhood, with its overtones of wholeness. That emphasis, consistent with the holism of the biblical writers, insures that we value *every* aspect of human existence rather than just the bodily/material or the mental/spiritual aspects—depending on our predilection. Insofar as God values every dimension of human existence, our perspective must be equally broad. It must take account of the needs of the body as much as the demands of the "soul"; it must be concerned with the manual aspects of life as much as the mental; it must respect the whole person.

We admit that the approach adopted here leaves us with difficulties. It does not account for the "intermediate state" of the Christian after death and prior to the resurrection. It leaves unanswered the problem of the Christian's identity during that period. Nevertheless, it seeks to take seriously the body in the context of God's purposes for people. This is implicit in the biblical statement that human beings are created in the image and likeness of God (Gen. 1:26-27; 5:1; 9:6; 1 Cor. 11:7; Col. 3:10; Jas. 3:9). The personal relationship which humans can have with God through Jesus Christ and the desire God has to communicate with them set human beings apart from all other creatures. What is astounding is that these are created beings who come from the dust and will one day return to the dust: finite, limited beings at home in the natural world. And yet, human beings are not truly at home in the natural world; they are spiritual as well as biological. Human beings are persons, and to live out God's image in us is to exercise to the full characteristics of personhood—making choices, holding values, being responsible for actions, yearning for love, developing meaningful relationships. To grow as full-orbed persons is to become more like God, and this is accomplished in Christ who was both fully man and fully God. To rejoice in the humanness of human beings and in the potential of personhood is to proclaim that humans are made in the image of God.

With our biblically consonant conception of personhood, we can turn again to human beings as they are known by neuroscientists and by ordinary people alike. We are physical beings; we *are* our bodies. We dare not ignore or underplay the valid data, yet we are aware that we are more than just our bodies. Experiencing *ourselves,* we realize we are conscious agents with hopes, thoughts, desires and needs (chapter 2). For Christians these data together constitute our perspective on the human person, a practical outworking of our holistic view. Stephen Evans stresses that Christians understand physical being in terms of personal activity, rather than the converse.

The hallmark of a Christian approach to human nature is that it accepts as the fundamental reality about individuals their existence and significance as an end in themselves. Our biological makeup, genetic inheritance, brain organization, early childhood experiences, interpersonal relationships, family responsibilities, spiritual awareness or lack of it, are all integral aspects of our activity and meaning as human persons. The total activity of an individual—particularly the activity of the brain—expresses what he or she is as a person.

That approach underscores the *responsibility* we must

exercise as moral beings created in the image and after the likeness of God. We are creatures with whom God can communicate and with whom God desires to communicate; we are beings loved by God and with purposes ordained by the sovereign will of God. Alongside the God-relatedness of each of us must be placed our vulnerability as living creatures. The interrelatedness of our body and personhood means that our personhood can never be isolated from the integrity (or otherwise) of our body and, in particular, of our brain. The human brain is a fragile implement, and when insulted in some way may have devastating consequences for the expression of an individual's personhood. The agony of the brain-damaged individual, presented in chapter 3, has been a constant undercurrent throughout this book.

The human brain, therefore, is to be regarded as a precious aspect of each individual, not because it encompasses all that the individual is, but because it *embodies* what the individual is as a conscious, responsible, moral being. The consequences of brain damage are consequences for the person as a person.

The fragility of the human brain is a manifestation of human finiteness. We are limited, because we are creatures in a God-ordered and God-sustained world. We must operate within a particular natural and social framework, which is not an arbitrary limitation but a limitation inherent within the Creator-creature relationship. A human being is not a god and there is no radical way in which we can transcend our creatureliness. Wonderful as the brain is, it is part and parcel of our finiteness, as demonstrated in our vulnerable dependence on its integrity. There is much of which we are capable, but also much of which we are not capable. The brain is complex, its potential is still to be realized, and yet it is so fragile. A Christian perspective accepts both facets of our existence; we recognize our dependence on God as well as the authority, responsibility and control bestowed on us by God.

Allied with out finiteness is our sinfulness. We find ourselves in conflict with ourselves, our neighbors, our environment and our God. We tend to abrogate our responsibility toward God by serving our own interests to the exclusion of those of others. Irrespective of the efficiency or brilliance of the human brain, it, too, is implicated in the human rebellion against God. Each human being is a unity, as much so in irresponsibility as in responsibility.

Human *dignity* is an aspect of personhood of profound relevance to the way we view certain issues, such as the nurture and control of the human brain. That dignity was bestowed by God in creation and redemption. All individuals are therefore to be treated as human beings with God-given dignity, regardless of their value to society or of their brain states. Human dignity rests not on what any individual can do, but on the fact that God loves all persons and Christ died for them. All of us, therefore, are under the protection of God's eternal goodness, having value in the sight of God. Moreover, dignity has to do with how we use our abilities, not with the extent of these abilities.

It is only within the context of the human being as a whole that the brain can be finally understood and its significance for human existence appreciated. Christianity affirms the significance of human beings and the meaning of human existence. In so doing, Christianity affirms the value of our fragile human brains.

# Bibliography

The following are the major sources of reference used. Where a reference was utilized for more than one chapter, it is listed under only one of the chapters. More technical references from specialized journals are not listed.

## Chapter 1

Blakemore, C. *Mechanics of the Mind*. Cambridge: Cambridge University Press, 1977.

Clarke, E. and Dewhurst, K. *An Illustrated History of Brain Function*. Oxford: Sandford Publications, 1972.

Eccles, John C. *The Understanding of the Brain*. New York: McGraw-Hill, 1973.

Nathan, P. *The Nervous System*. Harmondsworth: Penguin Books, 1969.

Rose, S. *The Conscious Brain*. Harmondsworth: Penguin Books, 1976.

Wittrock, M. C., et al. *The Human Brain*. Englewood Cliffs: Prentice-Hall, 1977.

## Chapter 2

Chomsky, Noam. *Language and Mind*. New York: Harcourt, Brace and World, 1972.

Descartes, René. *Discourse on Method and Meditations* (1637, 1640). Trans. L. Lafleur. Indianapolis: Bobbs-Merrill, 1960.

Dobzhansky, Theodosius. *The Biology of Ultimate Concern*. London: Fontana, 1971.

Gazzaniga, Michael S. "One Brain-Two Minds?" *American Scientist*, 60 (1972), 311-17.

Gazzaniga, Michael S. and LeDoux, J. E. *The Integrated Mind*. New York: Plenum Press, 1978.

Geschwind, N. "Language and the Brain." *Scientific American*, 226 (1972), 76-83.

Leakey, Richard E. and Lewin, Roger. *Origins*. London: Macdonald and Jane's, 1977.

Lee, P. R., et al. *Symposium on Consciousness*. Harmondsworth: Penguin Books, 1977.

Limber, J. "Language in Child and Chimp?" *American Psychologist*, 32 (1977), 280-95.

Popper, Karl R. and Eccles, John C. *The Self and Its Brain*. Berlin: Springer International, 1977.

Premack, D. "Language and Intelligence in Ape and Man." *American Scientist*, 64 (1976), 674-83.

Premack, D. and Woodruff, G. "Does the Chimpanzee Have a Theory of Mind?" *Behavioral and Brain Sciences*, 4 (1978), 515-26.

Pribram, K. H. *Languages of the Brain*. Englewood Cliffs: Prentice-Hall, 1971.

Sagan, Carl. *The Dragons of Eden*. New York: Random House, 1977.

Savage-Rumbaugh, E. S., Rumbaugh, D. and Boysen, S. "Do Apes Use Language?" *American Scientist*, 68 (1980), 49-61.

Terrace, H. S., et al. "Can an Ape Create a Sentence?" *Science*, 206 (1979), 891-902.

Young, J. Z. *An Introduction to the Study of Man*. Oxford: Clarendon Press, 1971.

## Chapter 3

Calder, N. *The Mind of Man*. London: British Broadcasting Corporation, 1970.

Ellison, C. W., ed. *Modifying Man: Implications and Ethics*. Washington, D.C.: University Press of America, 1977.

Gardner, H. *The Shattered Mind*. New York: Vintage Books, 1976.

Goldstein, M. "Brain Research and Violent Behavior." *Archives of Neurology,* 30 (1974), 1-35.
Henry, C. F. H., ed. *Horizons of Science.* San Francisco: Harper and Row, 1978.
Luria, Alexander R. *The Working Brain.* Harmondsworth: Penguin Books, 1973.
Luria, Alexander R. *The Man with a Shattered World.* Harmondsworth: Penguin Books, 1975.

**Chapter 4**
Adams, Jay E. "The Christian Approach to Schizophrenia." *The Construction of Madness.* Ed. P. A. Magaro. Oxford: Pergamon Press, 1976.
Burch, N. and Altshuler, H. L. *Behavior and Brain Electrical Activity.* New York: Plenum Press, 1975.
Chavkin, S. *The Mind Stealers.* New York: Houghton Mifflin, 1977.
Chorover, Stephen L. "Big Brother and Psychotechnology, I and II." *Psychology Today,* October 1973, pp. 43-54; May 1974, pp. 59-69.
Culliton, B. J. "Psychosurgery: National Commission Issues Surprisingly Favorable Report." *Science,* 194 (1976), 299-301.
Goldstein, M. "Brain Research and Violent Behavior." *Archives of Neurology,* 30 (1974), 1-35.
Mark, Vernon H. "A psychosurgeon's Case for Psychosurgery." *Psychology Today,* July 1974, pp. 28-33, 84, 86.
Mark, Vernon H. "A Psychosurgeon's Case for Psychosurgery." *Psychology Today,* and Row, 1970.
Montagu, A. *The Nature of Human Aggression.* New York: Oxford University Press, 1976.
Schrag, P. *Mind Control.* New York: Pantheon Books, 1977.
Smith, W. L. and Kling, A., ed. *Issues in Brain/Behavior Control.* New York: Spectrum Publications, 1976.
Spicker, S. F. and Engelhardt, H. T. *Philosophical Dimensions of the Neuro-Medical Sciences.* Dordrecht, Holland: D. Reidel Publishing Company, 1976.
Thielicke, Helmut. *The Doctor as Judge of Who Shall Live and Who Shall Die.* Philadelphia: Fortress Press, 1976.
Valenstein, E. S. *Brain Control.* New York: Wiley, 1973.

**Chapter 5**
Cantwell, D. P., ed. *The Hyperactive Child: Diagnosis, Management and Research.* New York: Spectrum Publications, 1975.
Claridge, G. *Drugs and Human Behaviour.* Harmondsworth: Penguin Books, 1972.
Collins, G. R. "The Manipulation of Human Behavior." *Journal of the American Scientific Affiliation,* 22 (1970), 8-13.
Gross, M. D. and Wilson, W. C. *Minimal Brain Dysfunction.* New York: Brunner/Mazel, 1975.
Häring, B. *Manipulation.* Slough: St. Paul Publications, 1975.
Hordern, A. *Tranquillity Denied.* Adelaide: Rigby, 1976.
Krupinski, J. and Stoller, A. *Drug Use by the Young Population of Melbourne.* Melbourne: Mental Health Authority, 1973.
London, P. *Behavior Control.* New York: Harper and Row, 1969.
Mascall, E. L. *The Importance of Being Human.* London: Oxford University Press, 1959.
Medvedev, Z. and R. *A Question of Madness.* Harmondsworth: Penguin Books, 1974.
Moberg, David O. "The Manipulation of Human Behavior." *Journal of the American Scientific Affiliation,* 22 (1970), 12-17.

Nahas, G. G. *Keep Off the Grass.* Oxford: Pergamon Press, 1979.

Schrag, P. and Divoky, D. *The Myth of the Hyperactive Child and Other Means of Child Control.* New York: Pantheon Books, 1975.

Snyder, S. H. *Madness and the Brain.* New York: McGraw-Hill, 1974.

Sutherland, S. *Breakdown.* London: Weidenfeld and Nicolson, 1976.

Szasz, T. S. *The Myth of Mental Illness.* Herts.: Paladin, 1972.

Whitlock, F. A. *Drugs: Drinking and Recreational Drug Use in Australia.* Sydney: Cassell Australia, 1980.

## Chapter 6

Berg, A. *The Nutrition Factor.* Washington, D.C.: The Brookings Institution, 1973.

Billington, R. *The Third World.* London: Inter-Varsity Press, 1972.

Cravioto, Joaquin, et al. "Nutrition, Growth and Neurointegrative Development: An Experimental and Ecologic Study." *Pediatrics,* 38 (1966), 319-72.

Heilbroner, R. *The Great Ascent: The Struggle for Economic Development in Our Time.* New York: Harper and Row, 1963.

Jones, D. Gareth. "Malnutrition and People." *Journal of the American Scientific Affiliation,* 30 (1978), 103-16.

Moberg, David O. *The Great Reversal: Evangelism versus Social Concern.* London: Scripture Union, 1973.

Mooneyham, W. Stanley. *What Do You Say to a Hungry World?* Waco: Word Books, 1975.

Morris, C. *Include Me Out!* Glasgow: Collins/Fontana Books, 1975.

Power, J. and Holenstein, A.M. *World of Hunger.* London: Temple Smith, 1976.

Rosenzweig, M. R., Bennett, E. L. and Diamond, M. C. "Brain Changes in Response to Experience." *Scientific American,* 226 (1972), 22-29.

Schneour, E. *The Malnourished Mind.* New York: Doubleday/Anchor Press, 1974.

Sider, Ronald J. *Rich Christians in an Age of Hunger.* London: Inter-Varsity Press, 1977.

Stott, John R. W. *Christian Mission in the Modern World.* London: Falcon, 1975.

Stott, John R. W. *The Lausanne Covenant.* Minneapolis: World Wide Publications, 1975.

Taylor, John V. *Enough Is Enough.* London: SCM Press, 1975.

Thielicke, Helmut. *Between Heaven and Earth.* London: James Clarke, 1967.

## Chapter 7

Brown, Barbara B. *New Mind, New Body: Biofeedback; New Directions for the Mind.* New York: Harper and Row, 1975.

Bube, Richard H. "Pseudo-science and Pseudo-theology: (c) Cosmic Consciousness." *Journal of the American Scientific Affiliation,* 29 (1977), 165-74.

Ferguson, Marilyn. *The Brain Revolution.* New York: Taplinger Publishing Company, 1973.

Fetcho, D. S. "Meditation: Do the Gurus Have Us in Their Grasp?" *His,* October 1977, pp. 1-6.

Forem, J. *Transcendental Meditation.* London: George Allen and Unwin, 1974.

Fry, P. and Long, M. *Beyond the Mechanical Mind.* Sydney: Australian Broadcasting Commission, 1977.

Fuller, G. D. "Current Status of Biofeedback in Clinical Practice." *American Psychologist,* 33 (1978), 39-48.

Haddon, D. "Transcendental Meditation Challenges the Church." *Christianity Today,* 20 (1976), 663-66; 713-15.

Hume, W. I. *Biofeedback: Research and Therapy.* Montreal: Eden Press, 1976.

Lee, P. R., et al. *Symposium on Consciousness.* Harmondsworth: Penguin

Books, 1977.

Lilly, John C. *The Centre of the Cyclone.* Herts.: Paladin, 1973.

Lilly, John C. *Simulations of God.* New York: Bantam Books, 1976.

Miller, C. *Transcendental Hesitation.* Grand Rapids: Zondervan, 1977.

Miller, Neal E. "Learning of Visceral and Glandular Responses." *Science,* 163 (1969), 434-45.

Ornstein, Robert E. *The Psychology of Consciousness,* 2nd ed. New York: Harcourt Brace Jovanovich, 1977.

Rigby, B. "Higher States of Consciousness through the Transcendental Meditation Programme. A Literature Review." *Journal of Chronic Disease and Therapeutic Research,* 2-21 (1977).

Sire, J. W. *The Universe Next Door.* Downers Grove, Ill.: InterVarsity Press, 1976.

Tart, Charles, ed. *Altered States of Consciousness: A Book of Readings,* 2nd ed. New York: Doubleday, 1972.

Wallace, R. K. and Benson, H. "The Physiology of Meditation." *Scientific American,* 226 (1972), 84-90.

## Chapter 8

Berkhof, Louis. *Systematic Theology.* London: Banner of Truth, 1958.

Brown, H. *Brain and Behavior.* New York: Oxford University Press, 1976.

Eccles, John C. *The Human Mystery.* Berlin: Springer International, 1979.

Evans, C. Steven. *Preserving the Person.* Downers Grove, Ill.: InterVarsity Press, 1977.

Gazzaniga, M. S. and Lovejoy, E. P., eds. *Good Readings in Psychology.* Englewood Cliffs: Prentice-Hall, 1971.

Globus, G. G., Maxwell, G. and Savodnik, I., eds. *Consciousness and the Brain.* New York: Plenum Press, 1976.

Hasker, W. "MacKay on Being a Responsible Mechanism: Freedom in a Clockwork Universe." *Christian Scholar's Review,* 8 (1978), 130-40; plus response by MacKay, and further contribution by Hasker.

Karczmar, A. G. and Eccles, J. C., eds. *Brain and Human Behavior.* Berlin: Springer-Verlag, 1972.

MacKay, D. M. *The Clockwork Image.* Downers Grove, Ill.: InterVarsity Press, 1974.

MacKay, D. M. *Human Science and Human Dignity.* Downers Grove, Ill.: InterVarsity Press, 1979.

MacKay, D. M. "Selves and Brains." *Neuroscience,* 3 (1978), 599-606.

McDermott, J. "I'm free because I know that I don't yet know what I'm going to do?" *British Journal for the Philosophy of Science,* 23 (1972), 343-46.

Myers, D. G. *The Human Puzzle.* San Francisco: Harper and Row, 1978.

Penfield, Wilder. *The Mystery of the Mind.* Princeton: Princeton University Press, 1975.

Skinner, B. F. *Beyond Freedom and Dignity.* Harmondsworth: Penquin Books, 1973.

Sperry, R. W. "Bridging Science and Values." *American Psychologist,* 32 (1977), 237-45.

Thorpe, W. H. *Purpose in a World of Chance.* Oxford: Oxford University Press, 1978.

Uttal, W. R. *The Psychobiology of Mind.* Hillsdale: Lawrence Erlbaum Associates, 1978.

Watkins, J. W. N. "Freedom and predictability: an amendment to MacKay." *British Journal for the Philosophy of Science,* 22 (1971), 263-75; plus a reply to this and other critics by MacKay.

Young, J. Z. *Programs of the Brain.* Oxford: Oxford University Press, 1978.

# Index of Names

This index does not include biblical names nor those found only in the bibliography.